Diverticular Disease

Dedication

For our families.

Diverticular Disease

Patricia K Black MSc, SRN, RCNT, FETC, FPA CERT

The Hillingdon Hospital NHS Trust, Middlesex

and

Christine H Hyde SRN

The Hillingdon Hospital NHS Trust, Middlesex

W

WHURR PUBLISHERS

LONDON AND PHILADELPHIA

© 2005 Whurr Publishers Ltd

First Published 2005
Whurr Publishers Ltd
19b Compton Terrace, London N1 2UN, England and
325 Chestnut Street, Philadelphia PA19106, USA

British Library Cataloguing in Publication Data

A catalogue record for this book is available from the
British Library.

ISBN 1 86156 446 5

Printed and bound in the UK by Athenaeum Press Limited,
Gateshead, Tyne & Wear.

Contents

Foreword

All who know Pat Black and who have read *Holistic Stoma Care* will be delighted to know that its success has encouraged her to undertake another book. Her expertise in stoma and wound care has enabled her to tackle another major pathology – that of diverticular disease.

Having qualified at the Hammersmith Hospital in the late 1960s, Pat Black served her apprenticeship as a staff nurse in teaching and district general hospitals in north-west London. Even as a young nurse her literary ability was recognized, with her publications of case reports and teaching articles.

In the early 1980s I was appointed to the Hillingdon Hospital, where I worked with my colleague John Sales. Having come from the same stable as John – St Bartholomew's and St Mark's – we were able to set up a Gastrointestinal Surgical Unit. We were fortunate to appoint Pat Black as a stoma therapist in 1985, one of the first in a district general hospital. Since then the unit has enlarged and developed, and in 1999 we were fortunate to be able to recruit and appoint Chris Hyde, to support Pat's increasing workload. Chris came to Hillingdon, having followed a varied career in both patient-centred and the commercial side of stoma care.

Over the years our two stoma therapists have also been directly involved with pouch surgery, liver resections and, more recently, rapid access clinics. They have a wealth of experience in the management of diverticular disease. This common condition of the western world can be treated by a simple resection, or can give the colorectal surgeon management problems when resection is complicated, leading to multisystem organ failure. Pat Black and Chris Hyde have been closely involved with the whole spectrum of care, but in particular that relating to the management of wounds and stomas. It is entirely appropriate that they should document their experience on the topic.

Finally, I should like to thank both Pat Black and Chris Hyde for their continued contribution to the working of the Gastrointestinal Surgical Unit at Hillingdon. They have become the focal point for clinic management, audit and the organization of a multidisciplinary team. I wish them success with the book, which I am sure will benefit coloproctologists and nursing staff.

Peter Mitchenere, MS, FRCS
Consultant Surgeon

Preface

Diverticular disease is one of the most common disorders among elderly people in western societies; early in the twentieth century it was believed to be extremely rare and a pathological curiosity. Burkitt and Painter, from as early as 1965, have written much on the subject, in which they called diverticular disease a 'twentieth century problem' and a disease of western societies. In contrast, diverticular disease appears to be rarer in developing countries. The prevalence of diverticular disease appears to increase with age and in western societies the reported frequency of diverticular disease occurs in different age ranges of the population; by the age of 50 years about 33% will exhibit signs of the disease, at 70 years 50% will exhibit signs of the disease and by 80 years 66% can expect to show signs of the disease. Fewer than 20% of patients will go on to develop complications, but these complications may be perforation, fistulae, peritonitis, strictures, bowel obstruction and haemorrhage.

The hypothesis about dietary fibre, or lack of it, has been perpetuated by many writers in human and animal studies (Brodribb and Humphreys, 1976; Findlay et al., 1974; Leakey et al., 1985; Manousos et al., 1985), many believing the disease to be the consequence of a low-fibre diet, as eaten in the western world. In searching the literature, with continuous regularity there are suggestions that fibre in the diet is beneficial in health promotion and disease management. Nurses are ideally placed to help patients understand issues of their disease management and effective promotion of health, but need to be aware of the guidelines and definitions of fibre intake.

We outline the history of diverticular disease and align this with the anatomy and physiology of the bowel, particularly looking at the function of the colon. The disease is then viewed from the uncomplicated cases and how best to look after the patient, to complicated disease, which includes three major complications: diverticulitis, haemorrhage and bowel obstruction. Surgery and its potential outcomes are discussed and a complete chapter on stoma care is included. We are both experienced stoma care nurse specialists in our own right, and Chapter 8 on stoma care can be used as a stand-alone section for the care of the patient with a colostomy, the rehabilitation process, the correct type of appliance to use and care in the community.

For many, having a colostomy, often undertaken as an emergency procedure, can be devastating and Chapter 8 endeavours to help the practitioner to think in a wider-ranging way and to consider the patient's culture, socioeconomic situation, beliefs, religion and any practices that may relate to his or her ill-health. Without understanding the culture in which the patient has grown up, the practitioner will have difficulty in understanding the reaction to the disease and illness, particularly when a stoma is formed.

Chapter 9 looks at literature from many countries around the world, both developed and developing, to compare the incidence of diverticular disease. Histologically, right-sided diverticular disease was the predominant pattern in far eastern countries, contrasting sharply with predominantly left-sided disease in the sigmoid colon in western countries.

As practitioners, most of us feel that we know enough about healthy eating and fibre in the diet because we have been advising people about it for many years, but fibre is an unexpectedly complex food fraction and a new fibre-oriented vocabulary is emerging that can confuse and misinform people. Chapter 11 helps to update current thinking, advising the practitioner of the new terminology of non-starch polysaccharides (NSPs) that are part of dietary fibre intake and the introduction of the dietary reference values and the Englyst measurement method (Department of Health, 1991).

Evidence-based medicine and evidence-based health care, aligned with research, can help both the promotion of good nursing practice and the understanding of failures in practice, with the aim of rectifying the situation. Nurses have an obligation to keep up with current literature in their field, read it critically and make balanced judgements about the quality and relevance of the work in relation to their practice.

Chapter 12 looks at alternative therapies and what may help and be of benefit to a patient with uncomplicated diverticular disease from Ayurvedic medicine to yoga. In Chapter 13 we look at consensus development in the diagnosis and development of diverticular disease. Importantly, in this chapter the surgical management is reviewed with regard to lowering morbidity, mortality and stoma formation, and who should be operating on patients to enable the patient to have the best possible outcome.

A glossary is included and a list of agencies that can help and support the patient who has a diagnosis of diverticular disease and his or her family.

Patricia K Black
Christine H Hyde
2004

The Authors

Patricia K. Black, MSc, SRN, RCNT, FETC, FPA CERT

Pat Black has been a Clinical Nurse Specialist in stoma care for 19 years at the Hillingdon Hospital NHS Trust. She undertook her Masters degree in Medical Anthropology at Brunel University in 1990. She has travelled extensively in eastern Europe teaching stoma care and setting up courses. She has lectured across the world on all continents at stoma care and colorectal conferences. She publishes widely in the nursing and medical press and in the national media. Her particular interest in stoma care is the patient who comes from an ethnic minority and the politics of sponsorship in stoma care. She is currently course leader for 'Foundations in stoma care' for nurses from non-specialist settings in association with Buckinghamshire Chilterns University College.

Christine H. Hyde, SRN

Christine Hyde came to the Hillingdon Hospital NHS Trust in 1999 as Clinical Nurse Specialist in colorectal nursing. She has worked with the multidisciplinary team and four years ago set up rapid access clinics for rectal bleeding and colorectal cancer. She has wide experience in the private and commercial sector in stoma care and has previously worked as a sister in a busy accident and emergency department; she then went to H.J. Heinz Company as an occupational health nurse. Currently she co-facilitates the 'Foundations in stoma care' course for nurses in non-specialist settings in association with Buckinghamshire Chilterns University College.

Acknowledgements

Writing a book is never as easy as it seems when the commission is accepted. Time has this strange way of suddenly running out as stress levels escalate. To the people who have supported us and stoically put up with us while we completed this project, we give our grateful thanks and apologize again for the days when we were cross and tired. There is no particular reason for the order of thanks, but only as they came to mind: Sue Rigg, Colorectal Co-ordinator; Robin Kantor, Consultant Radiologist; Barbara Stuchfield, Clinical Nurse Specialist Stoma Care; Sonya Francis, secretary to Mr Mitchenere; Juliette Fulham, Colorectal Practice Development Nurse/Stoma Care Nurse; Peter Mitchenere, Consultant Colorectal Surgeon and Clinical Director; Geraldine Gaffney, Head Nurse of Surgery; Bob Nye, Nancy Jackson, Paul Newman at Dansac, and many other friends who always enquired how the book was going. We are also grateful to Dansac Ltd for their support and encouragement.

Chapter 1
The History of Diverticular Disease

The written history of bowel-associated problems can be traced as far back as the Book of Judges in the Bible showing that the pre-Christian Israelites were well aware of abdominal injuries and problems (Black, 2000). But, even before the Bible recordings, the Egyptians in 2000 BC recognized disorders of the bowel, although writings often recorded on papyrus were not specific as to what these may have been. The Greeks and Romans were not to be left out in their writings on bowel problems; however, it was the Greeks with Hippocrates and Herodotus who made specific mention of bowel disease. Although Hippocrates is known as the 'father' of medicine (the Hippocratic oath) and is the most celebrated physician in history, little is known about him, other than that he lived on the island of Kos and taught medicine for money. He tried to dispel the idea of alternative medicine to lay the early foundations of biomedicine. Herodotus, although not a medical man, was a historian, who on his travels collected historical, geographical, ethnological, mythological and archaeological information recording wars and their causes.

After the Romans the period of time until AD 1100 was to be known as the 'Dark Ages' because it has been judged as a time in the western world of un-enlightenment and obscurity with political fragmentation and a lack of centres of learning. Yet, although the history of stomas can be traced as far back as Celsus in 55 BC to AD 7, quoted by Dinnick in 1934, diverticular disease was first described by Littre (1732) when he dissected a neonate and described what he saw in the bowel as a diverticular hernia.

In 1783, Matthew Baillie a Scottish physician who studied with William Hunter, succeeded to Hunter's famous anatomy school in London and in 1793 wrote the first treatise in English on morbid anatomy. It was within this treatise that Baillie mentioned diverticular disease (Oschner and Bargen, 1935). In the twentieth century Painter and Burkitt (1975) suggest that the history of diverticular disease can be divided into five phases:

1

1. The disease as a curiosity
2. The recognition of diverticular disease as a clinical problem
3. The recognition of diverticular disease as a growing medical problem
4. The surgical approach to diverticular disease
5. The role of the colonic muscle in the pathogenesis of the disease.

In 1927, Spriggs and Marxer suggested that the term 'diverticulum' originated from the word 'divertikel' which was said to have been used by Fleischman in 1815 in describing this anomaly in the colon. Between 1815 and 1869 many writers of medical articles were stating that they all believed that these 'divertikel' were not nascent but acquired later in life – thought to be caused by constipation. Even at this early stage in medical history, it was recognized that a fistula could be one of the associated complications of diverticular disease (Jones, 1859).

Although rarely seen in the nineteenth century, the recognition of diverticular disease as a clinical problem was emerging at the beginning of the twentieth century and was described as having complications such as fistulas, adhesions, peritonitis and stenosis (Beer, 1904). In the UK it was not until 1917 that the first 'classic' description of diverticular disease was published by Telling and Grunner (1917) before any medical textbooks.

The recognition of the size of the problem of diverticular disease in medicine was revealed once radiology advanced and could show that diverticula were not unusual; postmortem and barium studies were undertaken to demonstrate this. On the other side of the Atlantic, Mayo (1930) estimated that 5% of patients over the age of 40 years would demonstrate diverticula in their colons. This figure concurs with current postmortem studies undertaken in both Europe and America. Up until World War II, resection of the colon carried a high mortality rate of up to 10%. As a result of this high mortality rate, doctors felt that there should be preventive ways to stop diverticula of the bowel along with their complications and surgery. Believing that roughage could irritate the colon, Spriggs and Marxer (1925) believed that the bowel should be cleansed and there should be plenty of vegetables and fruit in the diet, but that any irritants from fruit and vegetables such as pips, stalks, pith and tough skins should be left out of the diet. As a result of the removal of these irritants in the diet and no other roughage, the low residue diet was born and recommended for diverticular disease with no proof that it would be of any value.

In the 1940s, when antibiotics were on the horizon, Smithwick (1942) advocated that resection of the offending colon with minimal mortality could be carried out, provided that the patient was fully assessed and prepared. Resection of the diseased colon then became a standard surgical procedure. In 1923 Hartmann (Black, 2000) had perfected the end-colostomy and this procedure was used and is still often used in many hospitals as a two-stage procedure for the resection of diverticular disease. However, in the twenty-first century a new consensus of opinion is evolving towards a single-stage procedure, although selection for a single or staged resection remains the most controversial issue.

The physiology of the colon related to the pathology of diverticular disease, which covers the fifth phase of Painter and Burkitt's (1975) discussion when they and Arfwidsson (1964) investigated colonic pressure in relation to the pathogenesis of the disease, and in 1964 Painter had suggested that the pain, often termed colic, that patients experience in diverticular disease may be caused by 'excessive segmentation leading to an intermittent functional colonic obstruction'.

Aetiology

The historical perspective on the aetiology of diverticular disease can be recognized as far back as 1853 when Virchow (Rankin and Brown, 1930) described inflammatory areas, particularly in the sigmoid colon flexures, as 'isolated circumscribed adhesive peritonitis' and in 1869 when Klebs investigated the relationship of diverticula and their associated blood vessels in the intestinal wall.

In 1930, Rankin and Brown were describing diverticula and their aetiology as a controversial subject, whereas Erdmann (1932) postulated that the presence of diverticula in the intestine was of no more importance than diverticula in other organs. Bell (1929) considered that multiple diverticula, i.e. diverticulosis, was mainly of academic interest. Mayo (1930) suggested that muscular weakness of the colon and not constipation or obesity was the underlying cause of diverticular disease.

Lockhart-Mummery and Hodgson (1931) suggested that after a certain age (45 years) the muscle sheath of the colon could lose its tone and diverticula result from the muscle weakness. Even at the beginning of the twentieth century there was wide divergence of opinion as to whether diverticula occur more frequently at the area of the intestinal wall where the bowel is weak, as previously described, or whether they are associated with the openings between blood vessels coming in from the mesenteric side, because, in the colon, diverticula present at any point along the circumference of the colon wall have added confusion to the understanding of the aetiology of diverticular disease (Rankin and Brown, 1930).

It was initially supposed that a weakened colonic muscle wall in obese people resulted in fat being deposited around the blood vessels, so making a potential defect in the muscle coat, although it was also observed that people who were thin and people who were wasted had colonic diverticula (Klebs, 1869; Edel, 1894). As no hard evidence could be found to support this hypothesis, obesity has been rejected as an aetiological factor in diverticular disease.

There have been many reasons postulated for weakening of the intestinal wall, among which are old age, muscular atrophy, fatty atrophy and even bacterial damage of the intestine (Henderson, 1994). Thinness of the colon muscle coat, enabling the mucosa and serosa to be in close approximation, is thought to be caused by excessive segmentation which is an acquired defect and not nascent.

In observing the history of dietary change and diverticular disease, Painter and Burkitt (1975) suggest that the British diet started to change from 1870. White flour with little fibre in it was available as early as 1800 and was taken daily mixed with rye and oatmeal, making a fibre intake of 600 g. As the development of transport and the migration of the work force spread around the country, and refrigeration became available, refined sugars within the diet became more freely available for all classes together with meat as a regular meal. Between the years 1860 and 1890 the intake of bread in the diet decreased and refined sugar intake doubled. Other than the periods of the two world wars, when there was food rationing, this trend has continued. If diverticulosis is caused by the move from a high-residue to a low-residue diet, it would follow that, about 40 years after 1880 and these dietary changes, diverticular disease would be noted to become more widespread, as in fact it did in the UK.

In looking at the cultural prevalence of diverticular disease, it has been found that there is a relationship between a population and its economic development (see Chapter 9) and industrialization. Painter and Burkitt (1975) suggest that it takes about 40 years for diverticular disease to develop within a community, after that community departs from its traditional eating habits, and that 'consequently the disease will not be found in a population until its diet and hence the quality of the faecal stream that its colons have to propel have been altered for about forty years'.

Painter et al. (1972), in researching historical and epidemiological studies on diverticular disease, found that they contained much circumstantial evidence to suggest that economically developed countries with altered dietary intake at the turn of the nineteenth century were more prone to diverticular disease. If diverticular disease is considered to be a deficiency disease, a deficiency of high fibre in the population's food intake, the answer must be to retrace our dietary footsteps.

The word 'diverticula' is the plural of the Latin word diverticulum, meaning a wayside house of ill repute. It was in 1916 that diverticular disease was first mentioned in textbooks in the UK and diverticulosis was first mentioned in 1914 (Painter and Burkitt, 1975). Although diverticular disease was little documented or seen in the nineteenth century, the few cases that were documented were accurately described by today's knowledge of the disease. In addition radiographic diagnosis did not become available until a century later. Painter and Burkitt (1975), in their historical overview of diverticular disease, suggest that the term 'divertikel' was used as early as 1815 by Fleischman (in Spriggs and Marxer, 1925). In 1859 in the *Transactions of the Pathological Society of London*, Sidney Jones describes a colovesicular fistula that was caused by diverticulitis and in 1870 Loomis (cited in Hartwell and Cecil, 1910) noted a case of peritonitis as the outcome of diverticulitis.

Chapter 2
Anatomy and Physiology

The digestive system starts with the mouth and ends at the anus. The tract would measure approximately 10 metres if it were laid out in a straight line.

The purpose of the digestive system (Figure 2.1) is to produce a chemical and mechanical breakdown of food:

- Ingestion: the act of eating
- Digestion: mechanical and chemical
- Absorption
- Defecation or elimination.

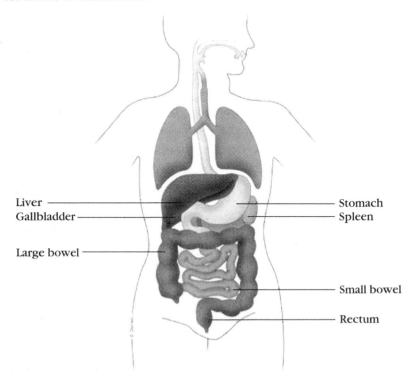

Figure 2.1 The digestive system. (Courtesy of Dansac Ltd.)

The digestive tract or alimentary canal is an epithelial lined muscular tube along which food passes by a movement called peristalsis. Peristalsis is a muscular action of dilatation followed by contractions as muscle fibres relax and contract (Jackson, 1979). This movement is not continuous throughout the tract because some organs store the food bolus whereas others churn and mix it with secreted enzymes. The food is then ingested and digested by various digestive juices and enzymes. Food is required to produce heat and energy for daily living and the food undergoes a complex process called digestion.

The enzymes that are secreted throughout the gut digest food. They convert the protein, carbohydrates and fats within food into their simplistic form, so that they can pass directly into the blood supply. The inorganic salts, water and vitamins are absorbed without chemical changes and waste products are eliminated

The digestive process changes as it passes along the alimentary tract. In the upper part of the tract it is predominantly under nervous control whereas further along hormones control the tract. The control reverts back to the nervous system in the rectum and anal canal. The food in the alimentary tract, along with a local nerve network, regulates the process of digestion.

Defecation or the elimination of waste products from the digestive process is triggered by the ingestion of food and the mass movement process of the bowel that occurs twice a day; both of these processes give us the desire to defecate. Control can be exercised to delay defecation. It is a process called toilet training, which begins at an early age and allows the control of elimination.

The Mouth

The food enters the mouth, the opening of which is protected by the lips. Food is bitten by the front teeth, incisors, passed to the back teeth, premolars and molars, to be masticated and chewed, and mixed with the saliva to form a bolus of food that will slide into the oesophagus through the action of swallowing.

The saliva is an alkaline substance secreted by the thought, sight, smell and taste of food through the salivary glands (experiment - think of citrus fruit and see if your mouth waters). With the aid of peristalsis (an involuntary muscular movement) the bolus of masticated food is propelled into the oesophagus. This peristaltic movement allows food and liquid to be swallowed together without choking.

The salivary glands are three pairs of glands comprising:

- The parotid gland: located in front and under the ears between the skin and muscle.

- The submandibular gland: located under the tongue.
- The sublingual gland: located anteriorly to the submandibular glands.

The salivary glands produce approximately 1 to 1.5 litres of saliva each day. The saliva mixes into the food with the action of chewing.

The parotid salivary gland produces salivary amylase, also known as ptyalin, which converts starch to simple sugar; the submandibular salivary gland produces salivary amylase and some mucus whereas the sublingual salivary glands produce a thicker version of mucus. The digestive process that happens when the saliva mixes with the food is instigated by the breakdown of carbohydrates. The saliva also has a cleansing function in the mouth, which allows taste buds to distinguish between sweet and savoury flavours. Saliva is rich in calcium and this is how teeth are protected from decalcification. The saliva is a lubricant that enables the bolus to be swallowed by making it moist; it also acts as an antiseptic.

Chewing continues until the food is manageable and moist; this is now called a bolus which is manipulated by the tongue and rolled into the pharynx. The soft palate closes the nasopharynx and the epiglottis moves to allow the food passage into the oesophagus (Green, 1978; Jackson, 1979; Tortora and Anagnostakos, 1981).

The Oesophagus

The oesophagus is a muscular tube approximately 25 cm long; it is designed to transport the bolus of food from the mouth to the stomach with the assistance of the mucus that it produces. The oesophagus passes in front of the vertebral column in the chest and through the diaphragm. It is positioned behind the left lobe of the liver and enters the stomach at the cardia. The oesophagus is made up of four layers, as is the rest of the digestive tract:

1. Mucosa: epithelium lined with squamous cells
2. Submucosa: contains blood vessels and nerves
3. Muscular: contains an inner ring of smooth muscle
4. Fibrous: dense connective tissue of longitudinal folds that contain the stratified squamous epithelium.

The food bolus passes into the oesophagus by the action of swallowing and then by peristalsis. It is possible to eat and drink at the same time and in a variety of positions from sitting, standing, lying down and huddled up in a crouched sitting position, all without choking as a result of the vagus nerve stimulating peristalsis. The vagus nerve is the tenth cranial nerve and is responsible for gut stimulation. The bolus of food has to pass over the larynx where it shares a common opening with the oesophagus. This is achieved by the tongue closing the back of the mouth, the nasal passage being blocked by the soft palate and the epiglottis covering the larynx as the bolus is swallowed. When this process fails we say that 'food has gone down the wrong way' and a cough reflex brings the food back. The swallowing reflex may be lost in anyone who has had a cardiovascular accident or is unconscious.

The food bolus takes between 4 and 8 seconds to travel into the stomach; liquid is much faster. The bolus continues along the oesophagus until it reaches the stomach via the cardiac sphincter.

The Stomach

The stomach is a J-shaped pouch with greater and lesser curves and ends at the pyloric sphincter. It is made up of the following structures:

- The cardia joins the oesophagus to the stomach
- The fundus is the dome-shaped part of the stomach and extends to the left above the cardia
- The body acts as the main reservoir
- The pylorus, is the last section before the pyloric sphincter

The stomach is made of three layers of muscle: the inner oblique muscle, middle circular muscle and outer longitudinal muscle. The stomach is a storage organ and is situated just below the diaphragm between the oesophagus and the duodenum; it is approximately 25–30 cm long and 10–15 cm wide at its widest part. The pyloric sphincter protects the outlet into the duodenum until the food is ready to pass as chyme. The bolus is mixed with the gastric juices which are controlled by the vagus nerve and the hormone gastrin. The motion of the movement of the bolus is to mix it with the gastric juices to change the bolus into chyme.

The gastric secretions consist of:

- water, mineral salts and mucus
- hydrochloric acid
- pepsinogen.

The vagus nerve and the hormone gastrin control the production of the gastric juices. The pyloric region secretes the hormone gastrin into the blood supply and it circulates in the body before returning to the cells in the stomach.

The vagus nerve

The vagus nerve is the tenth cranial nerve and the longest of the cranial nerves; its Latin meaning is 'wandering'. The nerve leaves the brain through the neck, into the thorax and abdomen. It supplies most of the muscles of the pharynx and soft palate. The vagus nerve enters the thorax and branches go to the lungs for bronchodilatation, to the oesophagus for peristalsis and to the heart to slow down the heart rate. In the abdomen, branches enter the stomach, pancreas, small intestines, large intestines and the colon for secretion and constriction of smooth muscle. Nerves in the abdomen and thorax join the left and right vagus nerves to ascend beside the left and right common carotid arteries.

The food bolus is churned and mixed with the pepsin and hydrochloric acid to form a thick paste that is called chyme. The mucus-containing food mixture is composed of partially digested foods mixed with the gastric juices. Every few minutes the pyloric sphincter passes a small amount of chyme into the duodenum. It can take between 2 and 4 hours for the stomach to empty.

Digestive enzymes

The role of enzymes is to stimulate chemical reactions in the food; to achieve this they require a specific temperature and pH.

Rennin

Rennin is required in infants. Its function is to curdle the milk ingested by the young child, which prevents milk from leaving the stomach too quickly, allowing time for the absorption process.

Pepsin

Pepsinogen is secreted into the gastric juice from both mucus cells and chief cells. When it is secreted, stomach acid instigates the conversion into pepsin, which breaks down protein into its simplest form of peptones. Pepsin requires a pH of 2 to work.

Hydrochloric acid

Hydrochloric acid is secreted into the lumen, which turns the stomach into an acid environment. The hydrochloric acid is required to activate the pepsin, so it too is required to digest protein. A hormone called gastrin is important in the control of acid secretion. Hydrochloric acid has quite a few functions:

- It provides an acid reaction needed by the gastric enzymes
- It is a solution for killing some bacteria
- It controls the pylorus
- It inhibits the action of amylase/ptyalin
- It changes pepsinogen into pepsin.

The production is controlled by the vagus nerve and the hormone gastrin. Gastrin is a peptide that contains 17 amino acids. The total amount of gastric juice produced is approximately 3 litres in 24 hours. Mucus covers the entire surface of the stomach to coat and lubricate the stomach wall, so preventing digestion of the stomach itself.

The intrinsic factor

The mucosal lining of the stomach secretes intrinsic factor which is required for the absorption of vitamin B_{12} in the ileum. Vitamin B_{12} is released from the ingested proteins through the action of pepsin and is stored in the liver. The failure to produce intrinsic factor causes pernicious anaemia.

The Liver

The liver is the largest gland in the human body and it is vital to life; death is inevitable without a liver. The liver is situated on the right side, opposite the stomach.

The liver weighs between 1.3 and 1.5 kg depending on age and sex. The liver is a very vascular organ which is made up of left and right lobes. It is found under the diaphragm, filling most of the right hypochondrium. If the liver becomes damaged by trauma it bleeds as a result of its profuse blood supply. A double supply of blood goes to the liver from the hepatic artery. From the portal vein, the liver is supplied with deoxygenated blood and the following nutrients:

- glycogen
- copper
- iron
- vitamins A, D, E and K.

In addition:

- The liver stores fat until it is required, then breaks it down to provide energy
- Urea is manufactured from excess amino acids
- Detoxification of poisons and drugs takes place

- Carotene is synthesized from vitamin A
- Antibodies and antitoxins are manufactured
- The manufacture of heparin takes place
- The liver is the main heat-producing organ of the body
- Synthesis of plasma proteins occurs
- Uric acid and urea are broken down from worn-out cells
- Prothrombin and fibrinogen are synthesized from amino acids (Jackson, 1979).

The liver has the ability to regenerate itself if needed. The liver supplies various chemical substances to the body via the blood supply through the hepatic vein. Waste is secreted via the hepatic ducts that form part of the common bile duct. The liver acts as a storage area for vitamins A, D and B_{12}. Harmful and poisonous substances absorbed by the intestines are stopped from circulating in the blood supply by the liver.

The liver produces about 1 litre of bile every day; it is stored in the gallbladder and enters the duodenum via the bile duct.

Bile properties

- Emulsifies fats
- Stimulates peristalsis
- Route for the excretion of toxic substances, poisons, alcohol, drugs and byproducts of red blood cells.

The Gallbladder

The gallbladder lives in the right lobe of the liver. The liver produces up to 1 litre of bile each day which is stored in the gallbladder. Bile is not absorbed into the blood supply The bile changes the chyme into its brown colour and the bile salts, one of which is amylase, are important for the digestion of fats.

The Pancreas

The pancreas is a lobulated gland 12–15 cm in length. This pinky-grey gland lies between the posterior abdominal wall of the duodenum and the spleen. It has a head, body and tail. The pancreatic duct lies within the whole length of the pancreas, terminating at the common bile duct where it meets the pancreatic duct at the hepatopancreatic duct. The pancreas produces up to one and a half litres of pancreatic juices each day; these assist further digestion of foods.

The pancreas has a twofold function: digestion and an endocrine function. The latter is the production of insulin and glucagon, which are required to regulate the levels of sugar in the body. Glucagon stimulates the conversion of glycogen to glucose.

Ileum (small bowel) (Figure 2.2)

Duodenum

The duodenum is the first part of the small intestine. It starts at the pylorus and ends at the jejunum; it is shaped like the letter C and is about 25 cm long and curves around the head of the pancreas until it meets the jejunum. The hepatopancreatic ampulla drains enzymes into the duodenum via a duct.

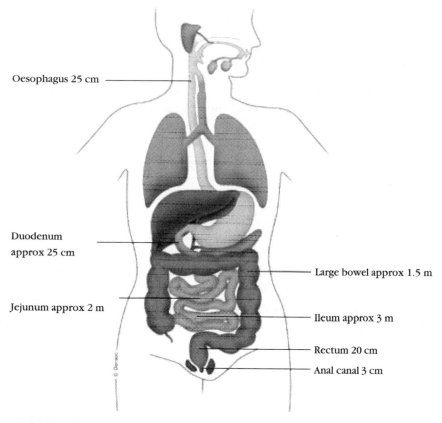

Oesophagus 25 cm

Duodenum
approx 25 cm

Jejunum approx 2 m

Large bowel approx 1.5 m

Ileum approx 3 m

Rectum 20 cm

Anal canal 3 cm

Figure 2.2 Measurements of the digestive system.

Jejunum

The jejunum is 2 m long; it is thicker and wider than the ileum and the folds are covered by finger-like villi. These villi contain a rich blood supply – they are the absorbers of the digestive process.

The Ileum (small bowel)

The ileum is a continuation of the jejunum. It is about 3 m long and has permanent circular folds (3–10 mm), which promote the mixing of the chyme. This enters the villi – the finger-like projections of the mucosal layer into the intestinal lumen.

Absorption of chyme is via the villi to the capillary and venous drainage of the gut. The remaining chyme, which is rich in bacteria and unwanted undigested food, enters the large bowel at the caecal valve.

The whole digestive process is aimed at processing food into the most simplistic forms that can be absorbed easily into the blood and lymphatic systems. About 90% of this absorption takes place in the small intestine. The other 10% is absorbed in the stomach or large bowel.

The Colon (large bowel)

The large bowl is about 1.5 m long, starting with the caecum and ending at the rectum. The caecum starts at the ileocaecal valve, which acts as a one-way valve to stop the reflux of bacteria from the colon into the small bowel.

The colon proceeds into the ascending colon, which passes up the right-hand side of the abdomen to the lower edge of the liver at the hepatic flexure. The transverse colon crosses from right to left across the abdomen, and extends from the hepatic to the splenic flexure. The endoscopist recognizes this area of the colon by its triangular shape. The descending colon extends from the splenic flexure to the sigmoid juncture – about 30 cm. It goes down the left side of the abdomen from the spleen to the left iliac crest. The sigmoid colon is S shaped and 40 cm long (Jackson, 1979). The rectum is a curved pouch, 9 cm long in young people, extending to 20 cm in adults. The rectum extends into the anal canal and is controlled by internal and external sphincters, which control defecation.

Function of the large bowel

The main function of the large bowel is absorption, automatic movement, and the formation and excretion of faeces.

The chyme is very liquid when it passes into the large bowel; in the region of 500 ml passes into the colon each day. It is here in the colon that absorption takes place: mineral salts, vitamins and some drugs are absorbed, along with 90% of the water content of the chyme. The large bowel propels the residue towards the rectum where it is stored. The large bowel motility comprises mass movement and peristalsis.

There are usually three or four mass movements during the day, which prompt defecation. A strong force occurs in the transverse colon pushing the chyme towards the rectum. This movement is triggered by eating and entry of food into the stomach, which is why the urge to produce a stool frequently happens either following a meal or during a meal.

Defecation is a voluntary act involving the brain, brain stem and spinal cord. The usually empty rectum fills; nerve endings are stretched by the contents of the sigmoid colon, causing involuntary contractions of the muscle of the rectum and relaxation of the internal anal sphincter; the voluntary external sphincter completes the process. In babies the act is an autonomic response until they are 12–18 months of age when the external anal sphincter comes under voluntary control.

The large bowel is heavily colonized by certain types of bacteria:

- *Escherichia coli*
- *Enterobacter aerogenes*
- *Streptococcus faecalis*
- *Clostridium perfringens.*

Bacterial colonization happens within the first week of life from swallowed bacteria and maternal contaminations. The colon is sterile for the first week of life (Society of Gastroenterology Nurses and Associates, 1998). Bacteria in the bowel are either harmful or helpful. If the bacteria are harmful they may cause diarrhoea; however, the helpful bacteria in the gut provide vitamins, mainly in the B group. A number of antibiotics, if taken frequently or in large doses, kill the helpful bacteria, again giving rise to diarrhoea (Green, 1978). The bowel maintains a flora of useful bacteria that are needed in digestion.

The Rectum

The rectum is the final 20 cm of the digestive tract and the final 3 cm of this is known as the anal canal. The rectum can accommodate about 400 ml of stool.

The anal canal ends with the anus, which has two sphincters: the internal sphincter of smooth muscle and the external sphincter, which is made up of skeletal muscle. The anal canal is lined by mucosal epithelium above the anal verge and squamous epithelium below. The anus is kept closed, except for the action of defecation, by the tone of the external sphincter. In some people, however, for a variety of reasons the sphincter loses its tone and can become weak resulting in incontinence.

Anatomy and physiology of diverticular disease

Diverticular disease is a twentieth century disease that results in part from changes in diet, age and lifestyle although there is little research to support this (Bassotti et al., 2003). It is one of the most frequent diseases seen in gastroenterology departments.

Diverticula are small herniations in the bowel wall; they can occur anywhere in the bowel. The diverticular pouches usually appear in the descending and sigmoid colon (Stollman and Rashkin, 1999), frequently manifesting at the weakest point in the colonic wall where the blood vessels supply the mucosa in the circular muscle layer. A diverticulum is an outpouching of the mucosa of the lining of the bowel. Diverticulosis is the name give to this manifestation and most patients with these diverticula will not have any symptoms. The symptoms of diverticular disease in westernised countries usually relate to the sigmoid colon. Right-sided diverticular disease is more prevalent in the eastern countries of the world. In countries where the diet is high in fibre and very low in refined carbohydrates, diverticular disease is virtually unknown (Hyde, 2003).

The outpouches are blind ends within the bowel wall where undigested food particles, faecal matter and debris can collect and become trapped; this can lead to inflammation and then to diverticulitis. The diverticular pouches usually appear in the descending and sigmoid colon; they can be a single diverticulum or in abundance. Sigmoid diverticular disease is common in the western world and thought to be caused by lack of fibre (Painter and Burkitt, 1975) and over-refined carbohydrates and flour (Keighley and Williams, 1997) in the diet.

Changes in lifestyle and eating patterns in the latter half of the twentieth century are thought to have contributed to the increase in diverticular disease. Another cause of diverticular disease is a consequence of high intraluminal pressure in the bowel, together with slow transit times of the stool. Stollman and Rashkin (1999) say that:

> High intraluminal pressure is caused by segmental contractions of the circular muscles and by contractions of the colonic wall between these segments.

Slow transit time of the stool is the time that the faecal matter takes to navigate the colon. This can assist the formation of the diverticula, which under pressure bulge at their weakest points. Fibre helps to speed this process but, as already stated, the diet is now lacking adequate amounts of fibre to accomplish this. The faecal matter stays in the colon for longer periods of time and becomes more constipated as a result, causing more pressure and straining on evacuation of the bowels.

All of these activities can result in the formation of a diverticulum at the weakest point in the circular muscle layer, where the blood vessels supply the mucosa (Bassotti et al., 2003). The lumen of the colon is at its narrowest in the sigmoid colon and therefore comes under vast intraluminal pressure; together with slow transit time of the stool through the colon (Mimura et al., 2002), this causes pressure that is exerted on the bowel wall, causing herniations at the weakest point.

Chapter 3
Investigations

Investigations into the bowel pathology are many and will depend on the symptoms that the patient is experiencing. In outpatients they will include:

- history taking
- abdominal examination
- digital rectal examination
- rigid sigmoidoscopy
- proctoscopy
- haematology, including a full blood count (FBC):
  - Hb
  - erythrocyte sedimentation rate (ESR)
  - C-reactive protein (CRP)
  - white blood cell count (WBC)
- carcinoembryonic antigen (CEA) to check concomitant cancers.

Radiological Investigations

Plain abdominal radiograph and barium enema

A barium enema (Figures 3.1 and 3.2) is the gold standard for demonstrating the severity of colonic diverticular disease (Halligan and Saunders, 2002). The radiograph involves the radio-opaque substance barium being inserted into the colon as an enema. There are two different barium enemas: a single contrast where barium alone is used; and barium and air as a double-contrast barium enema.

The patient has to have his or her bowel cleansed and all radiology departments have their own method of achieving a cleansed bowel. Essentially, the patient will take the bowel cleansing agents 24–48 hours before the examination; there may also be an element of a low-residue diet

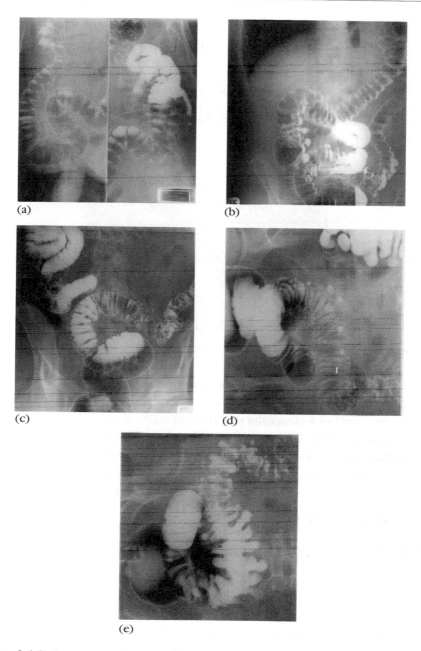

(a)

(b)

(c)

(d)

(e)

Figure 3.1 Barium enema: progress of barium through the colon, showing diverticular disease. (Courtesy of C. Bateman.)

included, with only clear fluids being allowed after the bowel cleansing agent has been taken. To achieve perfect views of the colon, there needs to be an absence of faecal matter.

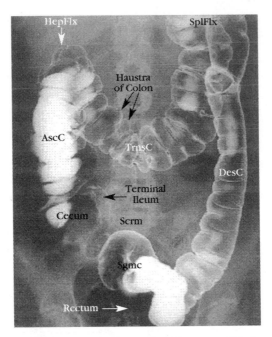

Figure 3.2 Contrast barium enemas: radiographs. (Courtesy of C. Bateman.)

In both examinations, once the barium has been inserted the patient needs to move around at the direction of the radiographer, in order to coat the wall of the bowel from the rectum to the caecal valve. It is important for the examination that the patient is able to hold on to the barium to maximize optimum pictures. A weak rectal sphincter will not allow this to happen. For elderly people this examination may not be pleasant because of holding on to the barium and the amount of turning that is required. The barium is a good medium for showing a bowel diverticulum. A barium enema does not allow for biopsies or removal of polyps. During the examination, if a biopsy or polypectomy is required, the patient needs to be referred to the endoscopy unit for further investigations. Unfortunately this requires more bowel preparation. It is possible to go from endoscopy to radiology but not the other way round, because of the barium.

Computed tomography

In the acute phase of diverticulitis it is important to have an accurate diagnosis. A straight abdominal radiograph is regularly the first to be ordered. This is followed by computed tomography (CT) if the results from the straight abdominal radiograph show that this is necessary. A variety of other abdominal radiological investigations is also available. The gastrogaffin swallow and follow-through or gastrogaffin enema is regularly used in patients who are thought to have an obstruction. This water-soluble medium does not cause harm if it leaks out through a perforation, because in time it will be absorbed. The gastrograffin may also help free the bowel from obstruction by increasing the water flow through the narrowing.

CT pneumocolon

The CT pneumocolon is, in the UK, becoming the test of choice and may be used in future plans of bowel screening for colorectal cancer. The rationale for this examination for the elderly patient is that it is kinder than the barium enema and the actual pictures show more of the internal structure of the abdomen as well as the bowel. The patient is still required to have the bowel preparation before the examination.

The CT pneumocolon is a procedure where air is introduced into the bowel instead of barium and there is no need to manipulate the patient. The patient is placed in the CT scanner. The disadvantage is that biopsies and polyp removal are not possible but, unlike with the barium enema, patients could have a colonoscopy performed the same day, thereby alleviating the need for further bowel preparation.

Colonoscopy (Figure 3.3)

A patient who has known diverticular disease may present a problem for the inexperienced endoscopist. The diverticula look like the bowel lumen but in fact are blind ends; it takes a skilled endoscopist to negotiate the diverticular bowel. The examination is usually one where diverticular disease is an incidental finding. The investigation is not one of choice in the acute stage because of the risk of the perforation with the endoscope.

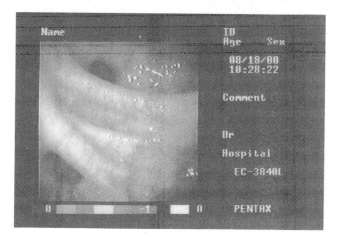

Figure 3.3 Colonoscopy showing a diverticulum.

Colonoscopy is a procedure where a flexible fibreoptic tube is inserted into the rectum via the anus to visualize the whole of the large bowel, the rectum, the sigmoid colon, the ascending colon, the transverse colon and the descending colon ending at the caecal valve. The procedure is carried out with the patient under mild sedation.

Colonoscopy is a procedure that is performed to visualize the mucosal lining of the bowel, to enable the endoscopist to take biopsies and snare any polyps that are seen, and to take photographs of the bowel whether a normal or abnormal mucosa is visualized on a monitor.

The procedure requires the bowel to be cleansed using bowel preparation, enabling clear views of the bowel to be obtained. All endoscopy departments will have their own preferred method to cleanse the bowel. Bowel preparation necessitates a method of cleansing usually in the form of a purgative and plenty of clear fluids 24 hours before the start of the procedure.

The actual procedure can be performed with or without mild sedation depending on the endoscopist's and patient's preference. Many patients are unable to tolerate the fibreoptic scope as it wends its way around the bowel, and sedation is vital for this group of patients.

Colonoscopy is performed with the patient lying on his or her left side with the knees bent up. A digital rectal examination should be performed first. The scope is placed into the anus and the flexible fibreoptic tube gently fed into the bowel. The endoscopist watches the procedure on a monitor and visualizes the bowel lumen as the scope threads its way around the bowel. The scope is made up of a main channel with fibreoptic capabilities; alongside this are two other tubes allowing water and air to be inserted into the bowel. The water tube allows the endoscopist to clear debris and the air tube allows insertion of air to open up the lumen and removal of the air. Biopsy forceps can be passed within the tube to allow the taking of a biopsy of bowel mucosa or to remove polyps.

The patient has his or her pulse and oxygen levels monitored throughout the procedure to ensure that there are no adverse reactions to the drugs or the procedure. If the procedure proves difficult or there is an impassable stricture, the patient can go directly to the radiology department for a barium enema or CT pneumocolon.

Chapter 4
Uncomplicated
Diverticular Disease

Uncomplicated diverticular disease or diverticulosis is a disease of the twentieth century that is thought to be associated with diet. Throughout the century, a fundamental dietary and eating pattern change also took place. Food is no longer a home-cooked meal made from fresh ingredients, such as meat and two vegetables, but something that has been processed and precooked with the addition of preservatives, taste enhancers and various other additives. There is a movement away from the tradition of sitting down at the table and eating; many meals are taken on the hoof and usually at speed. These changes have been the precursors of development of diverticulosis in our society (Keighley and Williams, 1997).

Age has been seen to be a predominating factor in diverticular disease in the western world; the older person does become more susceptible to diverticular disease (Bassotti et al., 2003):

- 40–50 years: 18.5%
- 60–70 years: 29%
- > 80 years: 62% (Keighley and Williams, 1997).

Recently there has been a tendency towards patients under the age of 50 developing diverticular disease, and deliberation has been that the disease was more aggressive in the younger than in the older patient. There have been several studies into younger patients with diverticular disease to determine a rationale for this development. Biondo et al.'s article in the *British Journal of Surgery* (2002) found that, in a total of 327 patients admitted to De Bellvitge hospital in Barcelona, Spain, 72 were less than 50 years of age. This research concluded that diverticulitis in the younger patient does not have a particularly aggressive course. In Houston, USA, West et al. (2003) found the same results – that the disease is not more aggressive in the younger patient. They also discovered that the number of younger patients did not reach statistical significance.

Symptoms and Treatment

Diverticular disease may cause only mild abdominal symptoms that are not of any real concern to the sufferer. Patients are reluctant to visit their GP for every minor ailment and the trend, today, is to look on the internet and fit symptoms to a disease or read a magazine's health pages. This leads to self-diagnosis and often self-medication; this can have a detrimental affect on the patient because he or she may incorrectly diagnose the symptoms and therefore take the incorrect medications. Other patients do not want to know what is wrong with them because, either they do not care or they think the symptoms too insignificant to warrant investigations; more worryingly, they are afraid that their symptoms are an indication of a life-threatening illness and delay seeking professional advice. This group of patients are the ones who may find themselves in the accident and emergency department (A&E) in a serious condition. Others will not have any consequences of ignoring their symptoms and will carry on with life in complete ignorance of diverticulosis.

Visiting the GP with vague abdominal symptoms may cause the patient anxiety, because the diagnosis may result in a serious condition. The GP has only an allotted time to see the patient, take the history, perform an examination and arrive at a diagnosis. Patients are not always good at describing their symptoms concisely and accurately when asked. Many patients are unable to name parts of their bodies when giving a history; tummy ache is usually a general description of abdominal pain without being specific to the actual location (Thompson and Patel, 1986). This can present the GP without a complete picture on which to base diagnosis and could result in the patient being referred to a rapid access clinic. These clinics have been set up to fast-track suspected colorectal cancer.

With the concept of the rapid access rectal bleeding clinic set up to diagnose colorectal cancer, investigations are colonoscopy, flexible sigmoidoscopy, air contrast CT pneumocolon or barium enema, all of which will diagnose diverticula if they are present in the colon.

In the asymptomatic patient who has attended the rapid access clinic with rectal bleeding or abdominal pain, with a preliminary diagnosis of suspected colorectal cancer, a finding of diverticular disease is a relief, until the relief of not having cancer recedes and the worry of diverticular disease impacts on the patient. These patients usually need reassurance because the term 'diverticular disease' sounds serious – an explanation of diverticular disease plus dietary advice to allay their fears.

Numerous patients with diverticular disease will be completely unaware that they have the disease. The symptoms are so mild that they do not cause any problems or produce symptoms. Most abdominal symptoms are often diagnosed as irritable bowel syndrome with no medical investigation being carried out. This diagnosis is often a self-diagnosed one rather than a medical one.

Investigating diverticular disease is twofold: the disease is frequently diagnosed as an incidental finding (Travis et al., 1993) while undergoing investigations to eliminate colorectal cancer or other colorectal diseases. The other means of getting a diagnosis is an emergency visit to A&E with symptoms of abdominal pain, haemorrhage or general malaise. These symptoms of diverticular disease will also require investigations to rule out any other colorectal pathology.

As in all consultations a detailed history is essential, especially with regard to the patient's bowel habit. It is necessary to ascertain the frequency of defecation, and the colour and consistency of the stools. Normal bowel habit varies from one to three times per day to once every 2–3 days; the way to determine bowel habit is to ask the patient what their bowel habit was before the current symptoms. The consistency and shape of stools are also important. To determine a diagnosis, as the stool may vary from hard pellets to watery stool, the following questions assist the doctor in the diagnosis (Bristol Stool Form Scale – Lewis and Heaton, 1997):

- Is the stool like thin string or thicker?
- What colour is the stool?
- Does it float or sink?

Rectal bleeding, usually associated with colorectal cancer, is one of the signs of diverticular disease and in the region of 17% of patients will experience rectal bleeding. Spontaneous cessation of rectal bleeding is common with diverticular disease. A minority will require hospitalization for their rectal bleeding because it can be profuse and constant; this symptom rarely requires surgical intervention (McConnell et al., 2003).

The patient who has symptoms of rectal bleeding needs to describe the type of bleeding:

- The colour of the blood: bright red, dark red or black?
- Is the blood seen on the toilet paper or in the toilet pan?
- Is there blood staining on their underwear?

Blood may not have been noticed; the patient may be colour blind or have coloured 'sanitizing agents' in the toilet. So other questions are required:

- Does the patient have pain?
- If so where is the pain?
- Is the pain constant?

- Does defecation relieve the pain?
- Does the patient complain of bloating?
- Is there a mucus discharge?

Abdominal examination is usually normal, although there may be tenderness in the left iliac fossa or descending colon. There will be a difference in the way investigations proceed from this point. Each establishment will have their own pathway for investigations from the 'one stop shop', 'nurse-led clinics' through to normal outpatient appointments. The authors' hospital operates a rapid access rectal bleeding clinic where patients are referred by their GP on the 2-week wait criterion. Patients are then seen in the outpatients department by the Consultant Colorectal Surgeon who will see them as described above, and perform digital rectal examination, rigid sigmoidoscopy and proctoscopy before referring the patient to the endoscopy or radiology department for investigations.

Radiological investigation will be a sigmoidoscopy, colonoscopy, barium enema or CT pneumocolon. All the investigations will show the diverticulum pockets if they are present.

When the diagnosis is confirmed, treatment for diverticulosis will be prescribed:

- Dietary advice
- Increase intake of water (2 litres each day)
- Analgesia if required
- Advice on bowel habit
- Health education.

There is additional advice on alternative therapies in Chapter 12. Patients need to decide for themselves the best treatment for their diverticulosis. Diet is very emotive and increasing fibre intake in some makes the symptoms worse. Through allowing the patient easy access to the colorectal nurse specialist by telephone contact, patients will learn how to control their symptoms so that they do not impose restrictions on their everyday activities. Regular outpatient appointments, once diagnosis is confirmed, will depend on local hospital policy. The author's hospital maintains contact with the patients through the colorectal nurse and this is found to be beneficial to all. Unnecessary outpatient appointments are reduced but contact is maintained. Patients appear to be pleased with this regimen. If there is a recurrence of their symptoms, help and advice are a phone call away. For the patient for whom surgery becomes the only option, the contact with the colorectal nurse is invaluable. The patient is more relaxed on admission because he or she will be fully informed of the outcomes of surgery, and the contact continues after discharge.

Chapter 5
Complicated Diverticular Disease

Diverticulitis

The patient with symptoms of diverticulosis may progress into acute diverticulitis. He or she may have experienced several episodes of diverticulosis before this change or, equally, this may be the first episode. This disease is an acute inflammation and infection of the diverticulum, giving rise to symptoms of acute pain, fever and nausea, and necessitates hospital admission. Diverticulitis can also mean perforation, fistula or abscess. Careful assessment of the patient is essential at this stage. Occasionally the diagnosis is clear as a result of the clinical picture and findings; other times more investigations are required. A plain abdominal radiograph provises a baseline for subsequent comparisans. A barium enema is not indicated if there is a clinical picture of perforation and for the same criteria that apply to endoscopy. Abdominal ultrasonography may rule out female gynaecological and pelvic problems that can have similar symptoms (Ripolles et al., 2003). Computed tomography (CT) with contrast has been seen to be of value in diagnosing diverticular disease (Rotert et al., 2003).

Perforation and peritonitis may be the first indication that a patient is suffering from diverticulitis. The patient may have had severe abdominal pain for up to 1 week before calling the general practitioner (GP) and, when elderly, the patient may be found to be quite ill and debilitated at home. The GP will refer the patient straight to hospital with a tentative diagnosis of perforation of the bowel or obstruction and abdominal pain, with a query as to cause.

The patient will present in the accident and emergency department (A&E) in acute distress and pain; equally he or she may present with vague abdominal pain and may already have perforated. Another reason for admission to the A&E is haemorrhage. Blood loss from a bleeding diverticulum is often significant, dramatic and without warning (Keighley and Williams, 1997). When the rectal bleeding does not require immediate hospital admission, patients are sent to the rapid access rectal bleeding clinic to have the bleeding investigated in order to rule out other pathology, i.e. colorectal cancer. The most likely cause of the bleeding is an erosion of the blood vessel where the diverticulum protrudes through the wall of the colon. A diagnosis of the origin of bleeding is imperative to rule out other pathology.

The patient in A&E will frequently require resuscitation with intravenous fluids, intravenous antibiotics and analgesia. The symptoms of an acute attack of diverticulitis can be similar: of gradual onset or a sudden acute attack of severe abdominal pain. The patient may or may not have noticed any other warning signs of being ill before being aware of acute abdominal pain. These are the symptoms that will bring the patient to A&E, usually in the middle of the night. Krukowski (1998) suggested that the policy in the care of a patient with acute diverticulitis is to manage the patient medically for up to 3 days before taking a decision to operate, provided that the patient's condition does not deteriorate. With this policy there has been a marked reduction in emergency surgery during the past 20 years with very little disadvantage to the patient (Krukowski, 1998).

The patients will be treated medically with intravenous antibiotics, pain relief, a nasal gastric tube for gastric suction and intravenous fluids. Some patients, however, will require surgical treatment for a perforated bowel. The symptoms of a perforated bowel are:

- Low-grade fever or a high temperature
- Raised white blood cell count (WBC)
- Nausea and vomiting
- Change in bowel habit
- Urinary symptoms associated with irritation of the bladder from the inflamed sigmoid colon near to the bladder
- A very ill patient.

Diagnosis of the diverticulitis will require investigations to differentiate from other problems, including appendicitis and colonic carcinoma. Physical examination by the doctor will show an absence of or dull bowel sounds in acute diverticulitis, localized left iliac fossa tenderness, and a palpable mass may be felt. On digital rectal examination a mass may be felt or tenderness noted.

In the acute phase of diverticulitis it is important to have an accurate diagnosis. A straight abdominal radiograph is the first investigation to be ordered. Blood tests are important, because they will show a low haemoglobin or raised WBC.

This is then followed by CT if the results from the straight abdominal radiograph show this to be necessary. A variety of other abdominal radiological investigations is also available. The gastrograffin enema is occasionally used in patients who are diagnosed as being in abdominal obstruction. This water-soluble medium does not cause harm to the patient if it leaks out through a perforation, because it will be absorbed in time. The gastrograffin also may help free the bowel from its obstruction by increasing the water flow through the narrowing.

The pneumocolon CT is currently being used at the authors' hospital. The rationale for this examination for the elderly patient is that it is kinder than the barium enema and the actual images show more of the internal structure of the abdomen as well as the bowel. The patient is still required to have the bowel preparation before the examination.

The procedure of pneumocolon introduces air into the bowel instead of barium, and there is no need for the manipulation of the patient to view the bowel or coat the lining with medium. The patient is placed in the CT scanner; it is a safe and accurate method of diagnosis for perforation or diverticular mass. The disadvantage is that biopsies and polyp removal are not possible but, unlike with the barium enema, patients could have a colonoscopy performed the same day, thereby alleviating the need for further bowel preparation.

Endoscopy in the acute phase of diverticulitis is not recommended because of the high risk of perforation. The endoscopy can be performed at a later date in the non-acute patient who, although there is still at risk of perforation, is at a lesser risk.

Complicated Diverticulitis

The patient with complicated diverticulitis may have:

* abscess
* obstruction
* perforation with peritonitis
* fistula
* mass.

Peritonitis can further be assessed as:

* purulent peritonitis
* faecal peritonitis.

Fistulae can be further described as:

* colovesical
* colovaginal
* enteroenteric.

Chapter 6
Case Studies

Case 1

This case study demonstrates how an episode of diverticulitis developed and eventually resulted in surgery.

James was a 48-year-old man who lived with his wife and two grown-up children. He was a plumber by trade with his own company. James was first admitted to hospital with an episode of acute diverticulitis about 6 months before he eventually had surgery. On James's first admission his symptoms of abdominal pain, fever, nausea and change in bowel habit resolved in 3 days with the administration of broad-spectrum antibiotics and intravenous fluids. He experienced three more episodes during the following 8 months, although none of these required admission into hospital.

Following James's only admission to hospital, he and his wife had a consultation with the colorectal nurse specialist (CNS) to discuss his diagnosis of diverticular disease. The CNS had explained about the aetiology of the diverticula, how they are thought to arise and the long-term outcomes. Ivy, James's wife, asked about diet and what change she should be making to their eating habits. The CNS explained to them that increasing their intake of fibre was said to be of benefit; however, they should not increase their intake suddenly but adopt a slow gradual increase over about 6 weeks (see Chapter 10). Increasing the intake of fibre will not cure the diverticula but can help control the symptoms. Diet and an increase in fluid intake are important to help control the symptoms of diverticular disease, but there is no cure; once the diverticula are present in the bowel, they are there to stay. The CNS also gave them written literature about the symptoms, and useful tips and advice on controlling the symptoms. The CNS also gave James contact telephone numbers in case he needed any more advice.

James did indeed telephone the CNS several times during the next few months either for advice or to report an episode of pain that had required his

GP to prescribe antibiotics. James also had a number of consultations in the outpatients' department to discuss his condition and to plan for admission for surgery. The consultant colorectal surgeon had, together with James, concluded that a planned operation would be in James's best interest.

This was the reason for James's current admission; he was due to have anterior resection to remove the area of his colon affected by the diverticular disease. He was admitted to the colorectal ward and, after routine admission observations and investigations by the colorectal team, he was seen by the CNS. The rationale for seeing the CNS at this stage was to clarify the preoperative, postoperative and operative procedures. The CNS explained with the support of a diagram, showing James the part of his bowel that the surgeon expected to remove. The colorectal consultant had already explained the operation, its risks and its outcomes, including the possibility of a stoma. A stoma is one of the outcomes that the consultant always discusses with patients undergoing a resection of the colon, or colectomy. The CNS explained the need for siting of a stoma before surgery (Black, 2000) The CNS also explained the implications of having a stoma (see Chapter 8) and introduced him to the stoma care nurse.

James commenced his bowel preparation regimen; at the authors' hospital it is commenced at 06:00 hours in order that the patient has completed the preparation before the end of the day and is not in the toilet all night emptying the bowel. It is important for the ward staff to monitor the outcome of bowel preparation to check that the bowel has been cleansed. Failure to achieve a cleansed bowel can compromise the surgical outcome by faecal contamination. The day of surgery arrived and James was taken to the operating theatre for his surgery. James underwent a sigmoid colectomy to remove the diseased section of his bowel without the necessity of a stoma. The diverticula had not spread into the descending colon and were only in the sigmoid area. The specimen of colon was sent to the histopathology laboratory for analysis. This is a routine procedure to confirm the diagnosis and make sure that the specimen shows no other pathology. Depending on the histopathology laboratory's workload, this result can be confirmed either within days or up to 2 weeks later.

James returned to the colorectal ward after his operation and time in the recovery ward. He was sleepy but easily roused; he had intravenous fluid and a urinary catheter *in situ*. James's bed was now in the postop. section of the ward, near the nurse's station; he was being observed at regular intervals, having his pulse, temperature and blood pressure recorded. The nurse also checked and recorded the amount of fluid transfused and the amount of urine passed every hour; his wound dressing was also checked for any oozing of blood. The CNS also checked up on James's condition, as did the stoma nurse – to check that James had not had a stoma. The stoma care nurse would have been involved with James's care if his surgery had meant that the formation of a stoma was required.

The first day postoperatively for James included taking care of his personal needs, mobilizing him, and the authors' hospital regimen for postoperative care included James being nil by mouth until bowel sounds are present.

The resumption of bowel sounds indicates that peristalsis has recommenced and that oral intake can be restarted; this process can take 5–7 days to happen (see Chapter 7). The colorectal team saw James on the ward round and they explained the outcome of the surgery. James was pleased that he did not have a stoma. The team told him that his urinary catheter would be removed later in the week and they checked his wound dressing. The CNS also saw James to see how he was progressing.

On James's fourth postoperative day, his urinary catheter had been removed and he was taking fluids orally but he had not yet had his bowels opened. The team were pleased with his progress; his wound was healing and James was walking up and down the ward. The CNS visited James to discuss his progress and plan with him for his discharge. They had already discussed these aspects of his discharge and had made plans for return to work but had not set any dates. James was keen to know if the CNS had any idea when he might be discharged; the CNS said that discharge was dependent on when he had his bowels open and his histology results. James continued making good progress and his bowels were open on day 6 which coincided with the team receiving confirmation of the histology.

The consultant explained to James that the histology confirmed the diagnosis of diverticular disease and that there had not been any presence of colorectal cancer. The consultant said that James could be discharged and have an outpatient appointment for 6 weeks' time. James was very pleased with the news and telephoned his wife to come and take him home.

The CNS spoke to James and Ivy before he was discharged to remind them of everything that they had discussed about the next few weeks and to give them the discharge leaflet. James was reminded that he would need:

- To continue his pre-surgery diet of increased fluid and fibre to maintain his bowel
- To remember that his normal bowel habit may have changed
- Not to drive for 6 weeks
- Not to lift anything heavy
- Not to return to work before he had his 6-week check-up or saw his GP
- And that he could telephone the CNS if he had any problems.

James returned to the outpatient clinic 6 weeks later looking fit and well, eager to go back to work. He was not having any problems and was very grateful to the surgical team.

Case 2

This case study shows an emergency operation for perforated diverticulum.

Jane was admitted to A&E during the night with acute abdominal pain; she had been unwell for a few days before her admission. Jane was in severe pain; her pulse was rapid and she was cold and clammy. The A&E doctor had examined her, requested a plain abdominal radiograph and referred her to the colorectal team. The registrar from the colorectal team had examined her at the request of his colleague, the senior house officer. Their opinion was that Jane had a perforated bowel and needed an emergency operation.

An intravenous infusion of fluid was started and Jane was taken straight to the operating theatre where she had a laparotomy and Hartmann's procedure with an end-colostomy. Her sigmoid colon had perforated, causing peritonitis, and there appeared to be a diverticulum present. The specimen was sent to the histopathology laboratory for a histological analysis. The colostomy was not sited preoperatively but on the operating table by the surgeon. Jane was transferred to the intensive care unit (ICU) from the theatre recovery suite. Jane required careful monitoring for the next 48 hours. She had the intravenous fluid *in situ* and was prescribed a course of broad-spectrum antibiotics; a catheter was draining her bladder of urine and a drain was *in situ* in her abdominal cavity. Jane was intubated for the first 36 hours and then weaned off until she was breathing unaided. Her wound and colostomy were observed regularly. Her colostomy did work in the first 12 hours and then nothing else was produced from it. The stoma care nurse (SCN) visited Jane in the ICU, having been alerted to her presence. The SCN took Jane a holdall of supplies that would be required for changing the colostomy bag. The wound did not ooze and the dressing was not changed until just before her discharge to the ward.

On admission to the colorectal ward Jane was conscious and alert, although she still looked unwell. Jane was introduced to the nurse who would be her named nurse during her stay. The nurse placed all Jane's belongings into the locker, including the holdall of stoma care supplies. She then checked all Jane's observations, checked the wound and colostomy bag, and left Jane to rest.

Over the next few days Jane's recovery was uneventful, but on the seventh day the nurse noticed, when she was changing Jane's dressing, that there was a red area at the end of the laparotomy scar; the nurse reported this to the nurse in charge and documented her findings in the nursing care plan. The following day Jane was taken by the SCN to the bathroom to learn how to change her colostomy bag; when the stoma nurse removed the colostomy bag she noticed a big red area creeping out from under the wound dressing. The SCN took Jane back to her bed after completing the colostomy bag change and then took the dressing off to look at the wound. As she took the dressing off it became apparent that a small area of the wound had broken down and pus was oozing from it. The SCN took a swab of the pus and informed the doctor of this event. During the ward round the doctors looked at Jane's wound and requested that the sutures in the lower end of the wound be removed to allow the pus to ooze out. By the next day things had become worse; the open area of oozing was now throughout the lower half of the wound and large gaping holes in the scar were appearing. The wound had totally broken down and was now a large gaping hole at the lower end of the wound. Jane was very tearful and distraught at the sight of her abdomen and she felt that she had suffered enough without this indignity of her abdomen opening up. The SCN talked to Jane and tried to help her understand why her wound had broken down and how it would heal.

The SCN explained to Jane that her wound had opened up because there was infection present. Jane asked how this could have happened because she had been on antibiotics. The SCN tried to reassure Jane that sometimes this does happen, even though taking antibiotics. The stoma nurse reassured her that the wound would heal but it would take a little longer and the scar might not be as neat as had been planned. The way forward was to pack the wound to encourage healing and to do this regularly every day. The importance of healing must be from the inside to the outside; if the outside heals first the cavity underneath will break down again.

During the next 10 days Jane needed a great deal of support and counselling to help her come to terms with her illness and now her change in body image. Jane had only been ill for 3 days before her hospital admission and coming to terms with its outcome was taking its toll on her. She had not been aware of having diverticular disease, because she had never suffered any symptoms from it or been aware of its existence. Jane had thought she had a bug at first, or maybe appendicitis. When she had consented to the surgery she had not fully understood the full implications of the proposal because she was feeling so ill when she signed the form. All she wanted was to have the pain stop and she felt that surgery was the only answer. The SCN explained that the surgery could be described as life saving because Jane's bowel had already perforated and bowel contents were escaping into her abdomen. Jane said she did not like her colostomy and was afraid of it and she did not even want to look at it. The SCN explained that most patients who had a colostomy as an emergency procedure felt the same way. The SCN explained that the colostomy was intended to be temporary and should be reversed some time in the future.

The nurse went on to say that the important thing was to learn how to deal with the colostomy, change the bag as necessary, and try to recover from the surgery. After major surgery the human body has to have a period of convalescence to let it recover. Jane's operation and its subsequent problems were having an effect on her and, because she had been so ill, she was unable to cope with these problems. When she is feeling a little better she will be able to deal with these problems easily. Jane said that she felt too weak to argue and she'd wait and see; in the meantime she hated everything.

Jane's wound began to heal slowly and the doctors told her that by the end of the week she would be able to go home and the district nurses would be able to continue with the care of the wound. This news cheered Jane up and she began to think about going home. Jane lived with her husband and he was looking forward to her coming home, but at the same time had reservations. He was not sure how Jane would cope or how he would. The SCN spoke to both of them about the discharge; she explained to Colin, Jane's husband, that he would need to look after the cooking and housework when Jane came home, because she would not be able to. Jane said that she was not sure about Colin's cookery skills. The stoma nurse went on to say that Jane would be able to look after herself and her colostomy but not the housework or cooking. She would be able to 'potter' around but would tire very easily.

Jane's discharge was planned with the district nurse visiting daily to change the dressing; the SCN made a date for a home visit to check on Jane and her stoma care. The consultant would review Jane at her routine outpatient appointment and set a date for the reversal of her colostomy.

Case 3

Jane was admitted 3 months after her emergency surgery for reversal of the Hartmann's operation.

Jane had spent the previous 3 months at home trying to adjust to life with a colostomy. She had managed to some extent but had not ventured out of her house very often. Jane had put her life on hold, waiting for a date for her reversal operation. During Jane's last outpatient appointment the colorectal surgeon examined the wound, which had taken a further 4 weeks to heal, after Jane's discharge from hospital, and although she had a wider scar on her abdomen the surgeon was pleased with the result. The consultant explained to Jane that he would have to reopen the scar in order to perform the reversal operation. The consultant went on to discuss the operation and its risks and outcomes with Jane and her husband. He explained that the intention was to join the colon back together and close the colostomy. He did warn Jane that this could prove impossible, in which case she would be left with a permanent colostomy, but he hoped that this would not be the case. Jane said that she felt it would be worth the risk because she could not live with a colostomy for the rest of her life. The SCN, who was also present, asked Jane what would happen if the colostomy could not be reversed. Jane said that she felt unable to think about the possibility of life with a colostomy but undoubtedly she would cross that bridge if she had to.

Jane was admitted to the colorectal ward for her surgery. This time she was able to walk on to the ward and be introduced to the other patients and nursing staff in the four-bedded ward. Jane had all her routine observations taken and was left to settle in. At 06:00 hours Jane started to take the prescribed bowel preparation regimen to cleanse her bowel. Jane had not had bowel preparation the previous time because of her emergency status. The nurse explained the rationale for taking a bowel preparation and its outcome. Jane would also be having a clear fluid diet. The second sachet of bowel preparation would be given at lunchtime, followed later in the afternoon by a rectal phosphate enema to empty the rectum of any debris. The nurse looking after Jane considered the outcome of the bowel preparation and enema successful.

The day of surgery dawned and Jane was taken to theatre for her reversal of the Hartmann's procedure, which was completed without any problems.

Jane was returned to the ward from the recovery suite and her observations noted. Jane had an intravenous fusion in progress and a urinary catheter and two dressings on her abdomen, one covering the main laparotomy incision and the other over the now sutured colostomy site. When Jane woke up her first action was to feel her abdomen to check if she still had a colostomy bag and she was pleased to find only a dressing.

Over the next couple of days Jane had an uneventful recovery and was soon to be found walking around the ward. Jane was like a different person, confident, happy and very talkative. The SCN found Jane talking to another patient who had a colostomy; Jane was telling her that it was not too bad once you got used to it and no it did not cause any problems; they even swapped phone numbers so that they could keep in touch. The SCN thanked Jane for her input with the other patient and asked Jane why she had had the change of mind. Jane said that looking back it had not been so bad and she was so grateful not to have the stoma any more that she could think like this now. The SCN was not surprised at Jane's change of attitude; she had seen it before. Jane's progress continued well and when her bowels opened Jane began to look forward to going home.

The SCN reminded Jane that her bowel habit may not return to its preoperative state. The nurse also gave Jane her discharge leaflet about the dos and don'ts after surgery.

Jane returned to the outpatient department 6 weeks later. She was very well; her bowels were opened up to three times a day and she was planning a holiday, because she felt able to consider this now. Jane thanked all the staff and offered to talk to any other patients if the SCN thought that it would help.

Chapter 7
Surgery

Surgery is reserved for recurrent episodes, complications or severe attacks of diverticulitis, or when there is no response to medical treatment. Surgery in the form of a one- or two-stage operation is considered to be a safe and reliable option. Hartmann's (1923) procedure is a two-stage operation; in diverticular disease it is usually performed in an emergency for perforation and faecal peritonitis of a diverticular abscess or obstruction. The one-stage primary anastomosis is proving to be a viable option (Belmonte et al., 1996; Regenet et al., 2003; Zorcolo et al., 2003).

Elective surgery is performed for recurrent episodes of diverticulitis, complications or severe attacks. However, there is a trend to perform surgery as an elective procedure, especially in the younger patient, and in some cases laparoscopically (Bruce et al., 1996). Surgical treatment is usually necessary in 20–30% of patients with acute diverticulitis.

Indications for Surgery

- Infection:
  - recurrent diverticulitis
  - paracolic or pelvic abscess
  - peritonitis
- Perforation
- Sigmoid mass
- Fistulae:
  - colovesical
  - colovaginal
  - ileocolic
- Obstruction
- Stricture
- Major haemorrhage.

Emergency surgery is a laparotomy usually performed by the surgeon to ascertain exactly the extent and damage caused by the perforation. This is determined by using Hinchey staging (Hinchey et al., 1978).

Hinchley Staging

Stage 1: involves a pericolic abscess
Stage 2: involves distance abscess in retroperitoneal or pelvic cavity
Stage 3: involves purulent peritonitis
Stage 4: involves faecal peritonitis.

Abscess

The formation of an abscess is more likely in the patient who has had previous attacks of diverticulitis. The treatment for the diverticular abscess depends on its size and location, and the clinical condition of the patient (Hinchey et al., 1978). The patient's condition is also an indication of the severity of the abscess. The abscess that resolves with medical treatment will not necessarily become a candidate for surgery. Drainage may also be a solution and this can be achieved with the assistance of the radiographer using computed tomography (CT)-guided percutaneous drainage. Patients for whom drainage is not possible and who do not respond to drug therapy will require an operation.

Perforation

A patient whose colon has perforated and has faecal peritonitis presents as an emergency that will require urgent surgical intervention. The patient will first need to be resuscitated before theatre with intravenous fluids and broad-spectrum antibiotic cover. In an elderly patient resuscitation may involve other medical specialities.

The perforation means that there is a clear passage of faecal matter into the abdominal cavity, causing peritonitis. The mortality rate can be as high as 35% (Sher et al., 1999). The operation again can be a one- or two-stage operation, with a Hartmann's procedure (Keighley and Williams, 1997). There is evidence that a single-staged primary anastomosis can achieve good results without the need for Hartmann's procedure and colostomy (Zorcolo et al., 2003).

Fistula

A fistula is an abnormal connection between two epithelial surfaces. This results in infection spreading from one surface to another. The fistula can communicate between two internal organs or lead from an organ to the surface of the body. The signs of a vesicocolic abscess are air bubbles in the urine and dirty urine. The diagnosis of diverticular abscess requires investigation because other factors can result in a fistula, namely Crohn's disease. Surgery is the most appropriate course of action with a diverticular fistula, involving resection of the diseased section of colon, repair to the other organ and a primary anastomosis. Alternatively, if a primary anastomosis is not appropriate, a colostomy will allow the fistula to heal and the bowel to be rested.

Obstruction

Obstruction is associated not only with diverticular disease but also with colorectal cancer where the tumour obstructs the bowel. Usually the obstruction in diverticulitis is caused by a stricture; not all obstructions need surgical intervention and unless there is a clear clinical need the patient should be treated medically to allow the obstruction to resolve. This can be achieved by resting the bowel, intravenous fluids and nasogastric suction on either continuous drainage or regular aspirations. Histology becomes paramount in any surgical procedure for obstruction to determine the actual cause (Wong and Wexner, 2000).

The Surgery (Figures 7.1 and 7.2)

The laparotomy enables the surgeon to view the abdominal cavity in order to see where the perforation has occurred in the bowel. The CT should indicate the site of the perforation and the site for resection. The presence of faecal contamination can preclude anastomosis of the bowel and surgery can be a Hartmann's operation that includes an end-stoma in the form of a colostomy. This type of surgery is intended to be a two-stage procedure, because the colostomy, at a future date, will need to be reversed and the bowel anastomosed. The severity of the condition will frequently determine the type of surgery (Krukowski, 1998). In 2001, a study in Spain of the efficacy of surgical management of acute complications in diverticular disease concluded that resection and intraoperative colonic lavage and primary anastomosis provided an alternative procedure for achieving a one-stage resection (Biondo et al., 2001).

Recent studies in Edinburgh have shown that emergency primary anastomosis in left-sided disease can be performed with a low morbidity and mortality in selected patients, even in the presence of a free perforation with diffuse peritonitis (Zorcolo et al., 2003).

An emergency operation will frequently mean that the patient will have neither counselling from the colorectal nurse specialist about the outcome of the surgery nor the possibility of formation or siting of the colostomy. This

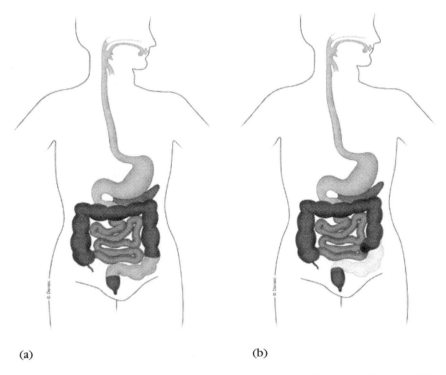

(a)   (b)

Figure 7.1 Hartmann's procedure: (a) before and (b) after. (Courtesy of Dansac Ltd.)

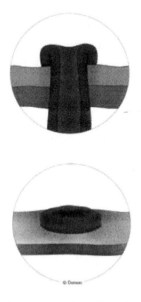

Figure 7.2 Colostomy: surgical reconstruction. (Courtesy of Dansac Ltd.)

lack of input can lead to postoperative problems in accepting the formation of a colostomy or an inappropriately sited stoma.

The lack of the preoperative counselling aspect can be overcome by the specialist nurse, but in a few cases a more formal counselling route may be necessary, such as a clinical psychologist. In the preoperative scenario a patient can ask questions, look at available literature or even meet a patient with a stoma. But preoperatively, if the patient is very unwell, all of this is irrelevant, because he or she will often say 'Do whatever you want'. It has been proved that a patient who is fully informed of impending stoma surgery will have improved postoperative recovery (White, 1997).

A stoma that has not been appropriately sited preoperatively can lead to problems in the actual management of the stoma (Black, 1994). The stoma, if sited on the operating table, gives a false idea of an ideal position. The table is hard, so creases and folds lie flat, and an assumption of where a patient's waist lies is all supposition by the surgeon. A stoma sited on the operating table is less likely to be in an ideal position and this alone can affect patient acceptance and the ability to cope with a stoma. A stoma that is planned is usually sited by the stoma care nurse specialist and gives the patient a chance to have input into the actual site. There is, however, a necessity to site the stoma within certain parameters (Readding, 2003) (see Chapter 8).

The patient with diverticulitis undergoing surgery is nursed on the colorectal ward and will remain in hospital between 5 and 14 days, depending on the type of surgery and hospital policy. Generally, patients will experience an uneventful postoperative recovery. There are a few patients who will have complications from their surgery, including:

- hospital acquired infection
- wound infection
- paralytic ileus
- bowels not working
- multisystem organ failure.

These complications will be treated in the normal way by the multidisciplinary team. The case history of Jane in Chapter 6 explains how one such complication was dealt with. Most patients will be discharged home with a definite diagnosis of diverticular disease and will not experience any further problems. They will have a routine 6-week follow-up appointment in the outpatient department and then be discharged.

Laparoscopic surgery

The current trend to treat recurrent episodes of diverticulitis with surgery is becoming more acceptable, especially in the younger patient, aged under 50 years. Many centres worldwide have adopted laparoscopic elective surgery for recurrent diverticulitis. This prevents the risk of complicated diverticulitis with perforation and the emergency laparotomy and Hartmann's procedure, which have a mortality and morbidity consequence. With the current trend of early discharge after surgery and the pressure on beds, an elective operation should produce a quicker turn-round than emergency surgery with its postoperative complications (Gonzalez et al., 2003). Laparoscopic surgery can be used for patients of all ages after the patient's assessment for suitability.

Laparoscopic or keyhole surgery is a minimally invasive procedure and recovery is therefore quicker. There will be a number of times that the procedure needs to be converted into a standard laparotomy. The rationale for this may be previous abdominal surgery that has resulted in adhesions, the surgeon may decide that it is not safe to proceed with the laparoscopic surgery or the operation may be technically impossible. The patient would require counselling from the specialist nurse about the surgery and the possibility of having the laparoscopic operation converted into a conventional one. The patient may also need to be sited for a possible stoma as a precaution.

The operation involves five or six small incisions instead of the usual laparotomy incision. These incisions allow the surgeon to insert the laparoscope and instruments to be passed into the abdomen. The surgeon would then be able to see what he is doing via the picture transmitted from the scope to a television screen. The surgeon is always able to decide whether to proceed with the full laparoscopic procedure once he has visualized the inside of the abdominal cavity.

The laparoscopic resection is not a faster method of surgery and one concern is the length of time that the procedure takes as opposed to conventional laparotomy. A study carried out by Dwivedi et al. (2002) concluded that the surgery time taken for performing the laparoscopic sigmoid colectomy was decreasing as surgeons gained more experience. The procedure was also seen to be a reliable and efficacious treatment with better outcomes for sigmoid diverticular disease of the sigmoid colon.

Reversal of Hartmann's procedure (Figure 7.3)

The reversal of the Hartmann's procedure is the second stage of the operation. To most patients this is the most important part of the whole process. The operation does carry risks and is not as easy and straight-forward as reversal of a loop colostomy. Hartmann's procedure involves

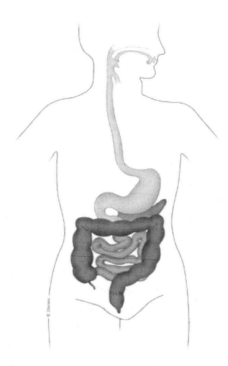

Figure 7.3 Reversal of Hartmann's procedure. (Courtesy of Dansac Ltd.)

another laparotomy and all the inherent risk associated with major bowel surgery.

One of the first remarks that the surgeon will make to the patient is: 'We had to give you a bag, but it's temporary and can be reversed.' The first question the patient has is: 'How long will I have the bag?' One or two patients believe that temporary means that the bag will be reversed before they are discharged home. A number of hospitals are able to give the patient a date for reversal of their colostomy. Unfortunately, this is not possible in most district general hospitals because of the restraints on bed availability and government targets. The reversal operation is not a life-saving procedure and, in the district general hospital, the patient is placed on the general waiting list.

The reversal operation (Keighley and Williams, 1997) is not without risk and will mean another length of stay in hospital. There has been research in Denmark about a fast-track rehabilitation after closure of a Hartmann's procedure from Basse et al. (2000). The conclusion of the study was that the inclusion of the multidisciplinary team after revision of the Hartmann's procedure reduces morbidity and hospital stay. Other hospitals are now performing laparoscopic closure of Hartmann's procedure which is proving to require shorter hospital admission (Sosa et al., 1994; Holland et al., 2002).

The patient's reversal operation may never take place; the patient may prefer not to have further surgery and be at ease with the stoma. Alternatively, the patient may have other medical problems that make surgery not feasible, or the patient may not be medically fit for surgery. Even though the intention of the surgeon will be to reverse the stoma, it may be technically impossible to reverse it and this may not be apparent until during the operation. The reversal of the Hartmann's procedure is not guaranteed and can leave the patient with a permanent end-colostomy.

The patient will need counselling from the specialist nurse about the nature of the surgery and the risks involved. The patient has to appreciate all the risks of an anaesthetic and surgery, as well as the specific risks associated with the reversal. Frequently patients put their lives on hold until the reversal operation, which involves not returning to everyday living, or work, and not seeing anyone outside their immediate family. This will place a strain on their lives and on their loved ones and impede their recovery. The ethos of this surgery is for the patient to return to their normal everyday living as soon as possible. In hospitals where a date for reversal is given to the patient at the time of discharge, a patient can plan and look forward to the future. The British Colostomy Association offers support, help, advice and leaflets on the reversal operation.

The operation involves reopening the old laparotomy scar, taking the colostomy back into the abdomen, and joining the proximal end to the distal end of the colon. The patient will then have two scars: the laparotomy scar and the scar where the colostomy was in the left iliac fossa.

After the operation to reverse the stoma, the patient experiences all the usual postoperative recovery episodes. The patient may experience a time of adjustment with bowel habit. It may mean that motions are looser and more frequent than before surgery or everything could revert back to normal. Some patients take a long time for their bowels to settle after reversal and loose frequent motions are a problem for them. Jelly babies and marshmallows (Black, 2000) work in helping to thicken the output if it is very watery. Incontinence can also be a factor after reversal; usually all these symptoms do settle eventually. Patients need to be aware that their normal bowel habit from before their original surgery has gone and a new habit will emerge. Most patients will recover very well and put all their anxieties of having a colostomy behind them and, for most, they will forget this period in their life. A few will still have problems: usually the length of time that it takes for them to recover and feel well again. Patients who have had surgery on their bowel still have access to the colorectal specialist nurse and will keep in contact if they have any worries.

The stoma care nurse specialist is the most appropriate person to counsel the patient with all the relevant information about reversal of colostomy and the recovery and convalescence period.

Complications of reversal of Hartmann's procedure

One of the main complications for the reversal of Hartmann's procedure surgery is the failure to reverse the stoma. A number of patients do opt not to go through the reversal procedure, some because of the risks of survival; others because they have accepted their colostomy and it has not caused them any problems. The author (CH) did have a 92-year-old patient whom the surgeons asked her to convince that he would be better off with his colostomy reversed. This man said 'My dear, why would I want to go through more surgery? When I go on an outing I don't have to rush to the toilet, my bag is convenient.'

Surgeons do appear to assume that everyone who has a stoma will want to have it reversed. Patients must be given all the options and allied risks, and be left to make up their own minds. For the patient who is desperate for reversal, this is not an option; they want their colostomy reversed at any cost. The patient who goes to theatre expecting to have the colostomy reversed and wakes up with it still there is in a desperate situation.

Patients have usually placed all their hopes and faith in having the colostomy reversed and never for one moment give any consideration to the possibility that it may not be possible. They are counselled at length about all the possible outcomes, but they do not appear to listen or remember that they may wake up with the colostomy. Patients feel let down and that they have somehow failed. These situations do not happen often but the possibility always has to be considered. At some hospitals this problem does not arise and colostomy reversals always happen. When the colostomy is not reversible for whatever reason, patients will require the advice and support of the stoma care nurse. Counselling these patients and offering explanations take all the expertise of the specialist nurses.

Other complications of reversal are wound healing. If the patient had problems with the wound healing after the first operation, the wound may take the same route. The stoma site can, in addition, have problems with healing. This can cause the patient emotional distress, because it will appear to him or her that the colostomy has reappeared. The patient will require wound assessment and appropriate dressing.

Another complication is the slowness of the bowel to resume its role of defecation. Patients often assume that, because they have been starved of food and drink, their bowels have no chance of working and do not appear to appreciate the importance of this complication. Fluid intake needs encouragement as well as diet. As a result of the fact that the patients have been starved, they become dehydrated and this is often the cause of lack of bowel activity. Most patients will have a bowel action by day 10. For those very few who fail to achieve this, it will be necessary for the surgical team to intervene for assessment. The first investigation will be a plain abdominal radiograph and then assessment. Surgery to address this problem is rare.

Chapter 8
Stoma Care

Body Image

The social taboos that surround body matter elimination are legion, so that, when a stoma is raised as a surgical procedure, as either an elective procedure or an emergency one, the individual's body image changes for ever. Stoma is derived from classical Greek meaning 'mouth' and is used as a medical term meaning 'artificial opening' (Black, 2000).

Body image, the mental picture of physical being that individuals retain, develops from birth onwards and continues throughout life; it is related to different factors affecting its formation and dynamics. A crisis such as the formation of a stoma leads to an alteration of body image and an awareness of the meaning of the change in appearance and function of an individual (Black, 1992). An individual's behaviour can be examined in several domains: physical, cognitive, emotional, cultural, sexual and economic. Feelings of violation of the body boundaries, degradation, mutilation and restriction occur. The intensity of emotional reactions to body changes is related less to the severity of the disability than to the assigned importance of the structure, and this appraisal depends, among other factors, on the individual's immediate social situation and past experiences. It follows that the importance assigned to the function will also be a determinant in the severity of the emotional reaction.

Many factors affect the patient's ability to adapt to an alteration in body image, and these are relevant to both the patient and the patient's family. These factors include, but are not limited to, the disease process, diagnosis, treatment, and medical and nursing care within the hospital and on return to the community. Most people feel that bodily elimination is a private function, managed best in one's own home. This can be related to the common notion that dirt is harmful to both the individual and others. In furthering the notion that dirt is essentially disorder and offends against order, elimination is not a negative movement but a positive effort to organize the environment (Douglas, 1966). By reordering our environment we make it conform to an idea. An individual with a stoma sees him- or herself as a person who has transgressed certain social expectations and failed in certain personal responsibilities.

Excretion and excretory behaviour are rigidly controlled in each culture and in each society, and in western societies there are strong prohibitions on the uncontrolled passage of urine and faeces. Prohibitions concerned with excrement are numerous, and it has been associated with madness, danger and witchcraft. To excrete through a different body exit requires a specific schema, which the individual and his society must understand if the individual is not to become a marginal member of that society. The western world enforces rigid laws in association with the civilized disposal of human waste by means of the private act of excretion, and the raising of a stoma can risk placing the individual in a liminal position as a person who may be dangerous to society. As human beings we draw boundaries between ourselves and the outside world. When these boundaries break down we find it profoundly disturbing, and when something in the system that we have conceived breaks down it violates something intrinsic to our sense of ourselves. Most people deal with this disturbance by denying what is happening. Littlewood (1985) suggests that, in western culture, if one can define oneself as sick when acts of excretion occur in the wrong place, they can be forgiven or managed in such a way as to ensure that the transgressor is not socially ostracized.

The individual who loses control over bodily elimination is presented with sensory phenomena (sounds, odour) that were previously within his or her control (Klopp, 1990). In addition to the person's own perception of these phenomena (actual or potential), the social perception of the phenomena becomes an issue, because of their very nature. We learn to control elimination at an early age, in private, so that exteriorizing the bodily structures that we use for elimination and loss of control over the accompanying sensory phenomena inevitably result in a changed body image. The change in body image after stoma surgery can be equated with a rite of passage, one that is not purifactory but prophylactic.

Following stoma surgery the individual's status within society is not being restored but redefined, and while being redefined passes through a transitional state that is deemed by society to be dangerous. After stoma surgery anxiety or even terror is expressed in relation to pollution beliefs. Although pollution beliefs are a cultural phenomenon, fear is exhibited by the individuals in understanding how they will be able to modify their behaviour and hide their stigma on their return to the culture and society in which they live (Goffman, 1963).

It is important to identify the specific areas most likely to affect patient outcome after stoma surgery. The most important area is the adaptation of patients to their change in body image, both internally and externally. In seeking to derive a framework it is necessary to consider the implications of stoma surgery. The sources of stress to patients admitted to hospital, especially those undergoing surgery, have been described by many researchers, among them Cohen and Lazarus (1982). For the patient undergoing stoma surgery, additional sources of stress arise: threats to body integrity, permanent physical damage, loss of autonomy and control, and the fear of the possibility of a histological finding of a life-threatening disease. Although profound distortions in body image are rare, there are many anxieties about the body and its image in relationship to its orifices, boundaries and bodily fluids. Stigmatization by exteriorizing excretory organs, especially later in life, may lead to an individual having problems with the re-identification of self or to the development of self-disapproval. This may be expressed in distortion of the total self, giving rise to confusion and negative changes in the individual's self-perceptions. People who had previously high self-esteem expectations, or those who take great pride in their appearance, care very much how others will perceive them and will find it more difficult to accept changes in body image and presentation of self. A stoma that is disfiguring to the body will be equally disfiguring to the mind. In addition, violation of the body's intactness can be perceived at a fantasy level as a physical or sexual assault. Kelly (1985) writes:

> . . . for the rest of the day I felt utterly wretched, sad and overwhelmed by a sense of loss and failure. I was not upset by the loss of my bowel *per se* but rather by the loss of its function. The sense of failure came from viewing my body as being wrecked by surgery. What really alarmed me were the physiological consequences, especially the incontinence and smell. These I believed would become the defining characteristics of my social identity and everything about me, my relationships, and the way others viewed me would be conditioned by these.

The major consideration in terms of adaptation to the change in body image after stoma surgery would seem to the length of time that the grieving process takes. Parkes (1972) outlined the stages that appear to occur in all individuals with a change in body image:

* Realization: characterized by avoidance or denial of the loss of the part followed by experiences of unreality or blunting.
* Alarm: characterized by anxiety, restlessness, fear and insecurity.
* Searching: characterized by acute episodic feelings of anxiety and panic and preoccupation with loss.
* Grief: characterized by feelings of internal loss and mutilation.
* Resolution: characterized by efforts to construct a new social identity.

In adapting to body image change after a stoma, Sutherland et al. (1952) were quoted as saying that an immense price is paid by the patient with a stoma for the cure and relief of the disease, which incorporates not only physical discomfort, but also psychological and social trauma. Devlin et al. (1971) looked at the effect of stoma surgery and found how devastated the patient with a stoma can be and how life could be quite complicated. Padilla and Grant (1985) suggested that there is a relationship between the quality of life and self-esteem among individuals with a stoma and that most stoma patients had positive perceptions. They suggested that individuals with poor psychological recovery outcomes would not return to their employment, would become reclusive and refuse contact with their social group and even their families. Wade (1989) indicates that a patient facing stoma surgery also faces the prospect of a change in appearance and loss of control over elimination.

Quality of Life

Quality of life (QoL) emerges as an important concept and outcome in health and healthcare practice and a perceived QoL is an important dimension of the health of both the population in general and the individual member of that population. The measurement of a patient's QoL after stoma surgery is an important focus in the evaluation of nursing practice. The role that nurses play in assessing and maintaining health will be one of the influences on the QoL of patients who have had stoma surgery.

There is much debate about what makes up QoL and health researchers and sociologists are divided between those who support a broad concept (Gill and Feinstein, 1994) and those who take a more pragmatic view (Guyatt and Cook, 1994). Even with debate and controversy among researchers there is a general acceptance that there are four domains to be examined when measuring a patient's QoL. These are the patient's:

- physical functional status
- symptoms and side effects
- social functioning
- psychological state.

When QoL is measured, instruments are used to provide information. These can be specific or generic. Generic instruments show a summary of health status, functional status and general QoL. Specific instruments will measure problems to do with a specific disease state, patient group and areas of functioning. The strength of specific indices is that they focus on areas that are most important to the patient.

Surgical interventions, whether elective or emergency, in diseases such as diverticulitis that will raise a stoma, result in psychological and physical trauma, which will impact on the lives of the patients involved, either temporarily or permanently. After major surgery, sometimes with little warning, patients suddenly find themselves having to adjust not only to the fact that they may have had life-saving surgery, but also to the management of an appliance that enables everyday functioning and excretion, and gradually have to learn to accept their lives with an adjusted expectation of normality.

Quality of life for a patient after stoma surgery for diverticular disease is what the healthcare professional is striving for. Nurses are continually striving to improve their quality of care and need information about the outcome of the care that they provide in order to redirect their efforts to areas where the outcome is not ideal. QoL assessment can provide such information and give a qualitative measure of the patient's subjective well-being and functional limitations. The data produced from such studies of stoma patients can be considered and used as an indicator of that patient's rehabilitation.

In selecting valid instruments for a QoL study it is important that the clinical questions are relative to care. The instrument should be:

- population specific
- suitable for both cross-sectional and longitudinal studies
- suitable for measuring appropriate health dimensions
- suitable for scoring and interpretation by care giver
- suitable for self-completion by all patients to whom it is administered
- validated against a 'gold standard'.

Patients who have had emergency surgery for diverticular disease and find that they have a stoma after surgery, often a colostomy, are devastated. Quite often, because the patient is being prepared for surgery as an emergency it may not be explained to, or fully understood by, the patient what the outcome of the surgery may be. Often patients will have no idea what a stoma means or even more specifically what a colostomy is. It is particularly important that this group of patients who undergo emergency surgery are identified and their QoL problems resolved.

There are many QoL indices that are available, but it is important that the correct index be used and often it is the functional limitations after stoma surgery that need to be measured. A suitable index is the one devised by Padilla and Grant (1985), which was developed to measure the QoL as an outcome variable in cancer patients. In looking at a QoL study for stoma patients other domains should be considered such as:

- psychological well-being
- physical well-being
- body image
- pain
- sexual activity
- nutrition
- social concerns
- patient satisfaction
- patient improvement
- patient experience
- self-efficacy
- help and advice.

These headings then form a basis for drawing up a QoL questionnaire to help the healthcare professional in the care of the patient with a stoma. One score per domain is entered, enabling analysis to be performed easily. The scores are 0 for the worst and 100 for the best QoL. From the questions a global score or index can be generated that gives the best overall information about the patient's well-being.

Often, in these studies, the scores show improvement in the patient's QoL after hospital discharge, and then a trend for stability over a long period. Time is not the only predictive factor of QoL evolution after hospital discharge. A close link has also been noticed between hospital discharge and patients' feelings about satisfaction with medical care, confidence in appliance changing and relationships with the community nurse, either the stoma care nurse or the district nurse. The more satisfied patients are with their care and information received, the better the QoL evolution.

Stoma Siting

The careful siting of a stoma, whether temporary or permanent, plays an essential role in the rehabilitation of the patient. In elective cases, whatever the reason for a stoma, it is usual for the stoma care nurse to site the stoma preoperatively and to counsel the patient about the possible outcomes. All this takes place in a far more relaxed atmosphere where the patient can ask coherent questions about what is going to happen to him- or herself. Often, in the case of diverticulitis where surgical intervention will be as an emergency, the stoma is not sited preoperatively because the patient goes to theatre for surgery via the accident and emergency department (A&E), often during unsocial hours. The problems that can arise from a badly sited stoma can include the patient being unable to see the stoma because of bodily protrusions, and therefore being unable to manage the appliance, causing leakage and sore skin. There may be retraction or prolapse of the stoma, or a parastomal hernia may occur.

In 1981, Breckman suggested that, before the advent of stoma care nurses in the UK, the siting of the stoma was left to the surgeon and was often decided after the patient had been anaesthetized, and at the end of the surgery. Yet, in 1989, Wade found, in her study of stoma care nurses and their patients, that very little had changed in the siting of the patient's stoma. As one ward sister in the study stated:

> It is usually done by the surgeon with the patient on the operating table, so you can imagine the problems that therefore result.

The stomas created in emergency surgery are often more difficult. They are always far too near the main wound site or far too high up under the rib cage, which causes difficulty once the patient has regained consciousness and sits up. In Wade's research (1989), one surgeon commented in his interview:

> . . . although the stoma care nurse sites the elective preoperative patients for the stoma, I always move it by a centimetre to assert my independence.

Although it would be expected that stomas sited electively would be easier to see and manage, emergency stomas did not fare too badly. In the Wade study, *A Stoma is for Life* (1989), of the patients who had stomas raised as an emergency, 81.5% stated that they could see their stomas easily compared with 86.9% who underwent elective surgery.

The importance of having a stoma sited correctly cannot be stressed enough (CORCE, 1997). For most caucasian patients the stoma will be sited below the umbilicus, but patients from ethnic minorities may need the stoma to be sited on a different area of the abdomen. If the patient is to have elective surgery, as some patients with diverticular disease do, after the decision by the surgeon has been made the patient will often be seen in hospital by the stoma care nurse who is a member of the multidisciplinary colorectal team. If there is no stoma care nurse, sometimes an experienced ward sister on the colorectal unit will site the patient's stoma. When first assessing the patient the nurse will mentally be taking in images of the patient's body and physique. The nurse will discuss with the patient his or her lifestyle, work and leisure pursuits. For patients who are working the nature of their employment is important, because the nurse should be aware if the patient is expected to do heavy lifting or work of a heavy manual nature. In situations such as these it is important to consider the planned stoma area in view of possible postoperative parastomal herniation or prolapse.

To site the patient, the nurse or stoma care nurse will require the patient to lie flat on the bed and expose the abdomen. The abdomen is examined for creases, weight loss indications, previous scars and bony prominences, skin problems and the natural waistline. If the stoma is to be a colostomy it will be sited in the left iliac fossa or, if an ileostomy, in the right iliac fossa. A small mark is placed on the correct side for the appropriate stoma. The patient will then be asked to sit up on the edge of the bed for the nurse to see if the mark is in the correct place for the patient to be able to care for him- or herself and to make sure that there are no rolls of adipose tissue falling over the potential stoma site and therefore occluding the stoma. If there are gullies or rolls of adipose tissue the appliance will not fit securely and leakage leading to sore skin will become a problem for the patient. While assessing the correct site, the nurse will be explaining to the patient what she is doing and why. Enquiries are made of the patient on what sort of clothes he or she wears, where the waistline is, and if a man where his trouser line comes and whether he wears braces or a belt. Many older women become concerned because they may wear a support girdle or pants. They should be assured that a hole can be made in the girdle for the appliance to come through. Patients who require a support girdle are allowed three a year on prescription and this is not just a prerogative of women, men may also need a support girdle if they do heavy lifting. If it appears that siting of the stoma may be difficult because of the patient's shape, the patient should put on normal clothes and the stoma site be reassessed wearing everyday clothes. If the patient is likely to lose weight over time after surgery, and it must be remembered that some will be lost postoperatively, the stoma must not disappear into skinfolds. Once the site of the stoma has been agreed with the nurse and patient, the nurse uses a skin marker pen to mark the spot and cover with clear tape to maintain the mark until surgery. Biro and felt-tip pens are unsuitable because they contain colophony which may cause skin allergies.

Areas to avoid in siting stomas

- The waistline
- Hip bones
- Previous scar lines
- The groin areas
- Fat folds and bulges
- The umbilicus
- Current fistula and drain sites
- Under pendulous breasts

- The primary incision site
- Any areas that have skin problems such as psoriasis
- Areas crossed by straps for artificial limbs or other surgical appliances
- Areas where, if there was weight loss or gain, the stoma would be difficult to manage.

At the end of the siting of the stoma, it should be recorded in the patient notes that the stoma site has been marked with the consent of the patient in an agreed area and the site on the body recorded either by diagram or by written word. In some hospitals stoma care nurses use digital cameras and place the photograph in the patient's medical notes. By recording this information in the medical notes, the nurse is covered if there should be any query or litigation about the site of the stoma.

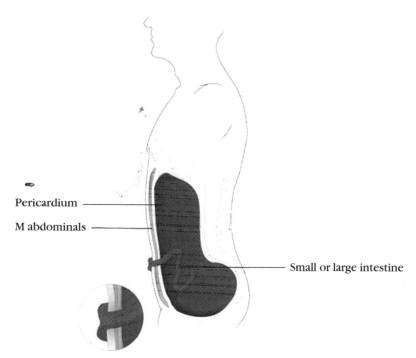

Pericardium

M abdominals

Small or large intestine

Figure 8.1 Ostomy: side view. (Courtesy of Dansac Ltd.)

Emergency Surgery

Patients who have diverticulitis may suddenly find that they have an exacerbation of the disease and an emergency admission to hospital is needed. After initial investigations are done the patient will be prepared for an emergency operation. It is often not the reason for the emergency surgery that is considered, but the implications of the sudden event that affect the eventual rehabilitation of the ostomate. Abrams (1984) has suggested that there is never too much time to prepare the patient for the outcome of surgery resulting in a possible stoma whether permanent or temporary:

> In my experience the worst results, psychologically, have been with patients who have either received no preparation or were too sick to be prepared or who were given inaccurate or dishonest information.

A significant proportion of ostomates undergo emergency surgery and Devlin (1984) suggests that about 30% of patients with a stoma fall into this category and that nursing and medical attitudes are crucial to the ultimate long-term effect of recovery for this group of patients.

When a patient undergoes emergency bowel surgery for diverticulitis, there is little or no time for preoperative preparation, let alone siting of the stoma. Many patients are admitted to A&E at night or in the early hours of the morning, and proceed to theatre from the department, going to a ward only on return from theatre. Many patients therefore wake to find that they have a stoma without either understanding or even knowing beforehand of its possibility. Morrison (1978) suggests subsequently that it is not surprising that many patients may feel that they have been assaulted or unable to accept a stoma to which they never agreed in the first place. It appears that the obstacles to rehabilitation and adaptation are greater for the patient who has emergency stoma surgery than for the patient who has elective surgery.

In interpreting the research about whether patients having an emergency stoma with little or no preoperative preparation fare badly as opposed to the elective patient who receives adequate counselling and information, it seems that those patients who know most about their operations have the slowest recovery. In the two studies by Cohen (1975) and Cohen and Lazarus (1973), which investigate the relationship between the recovery from surgery and the avoidance or vigilance towards seeking information about the condition and surgery, it has been suggested that vigilant 'copers' seek to master the world by seeking information, although this style is maladaptive in the postoperative period when patients are relatively powerless. In the current age when the internet is so readily available, many patients and relatives come armed with files of information about their disease and operative procedures before or after surgery, questioning the information that they are receiving from the nurses and doctors.

In Wade's research (1989) her second interviews with stoma patients revealed that, of her cohort, 26.9% of the women and 19.1% of the men said that they were unable to accept their stoma, with extreme negativity demonstrated by 6.7% of the patients. Acceptance of the stoma was higher among those with a permanent stoma, 81.5%, than those with temporary colostomies. One patient states:

> They never told me beforehand that I was going to have a stoma. The thing that worries me is the fact that I feel a burden to my wife. If I did not have this nagging pain in my legs and back – if I did not have that I could go out and walk about freely – I think you probably know the answer would be ok, 100%.

For those patients still with a temporary stoma 1 year after surgery, 27% of women and 19% of men still felt unable to accept their stoma.

Case study

John, aged 37, was admitted from his place of work to the hospital A&E department at 10am complaining of severe abdominal pain and nausea, tachycardia and sweating. He was examined by a doctor from the colorectal team who decided that John had an acute appendicitis and would be prepared for theatre immediately.

At operation an appendix incision was made but the surgeon quickly noted that the appendix was normal and proceeded to a midline laparotomy wound. In the descending sigmoid colon they found a perforated bowel significant of diverticulitis. The bowel was removed in a Hartmann's procedure resulting in a colostomy.

After surgery John and his wife were told the diagnosis and the colostomy was explained to them. They were told that the colostomy was reversible in a few months after John had recovered. John found this news of his colostomy very difficult to take in. He was a subcontracted, self-employed lorry driver and had little day-to-day access to a toilet with private facilities to cope with appliance changing.

John's psychological recovery in hospital was stormy because he could not accept that he had a stoma and would talk about his stoma as if it was not part of his body. He would walk around the ward with his pyjama top wide open and his stoma bag showing which could become offensive to other patients and relatives. When asked if he could keep his appliance covered while up and about he said that he always walked about with his shirt off and he could not see what the problem was as there was nothing unusual about his abdomen. The stoma care nurse was asked to try to help him by empowering him towards self-care, but John was very reluctant. Even with his wife's encouragement John said that his wife would see to the 'bag'.

Two weeks after his discharge, John would telephone every day to try to rearrange his postoperative follow-up and to be put straight on the list for reversal. He was seen in clinic at 8 weeks after surgery and was told he would be put on the waiting list for reversal. Two weeks later John opted for private care and had a reversal the following week, discharging himself from hospital after 5 days. So far John had not attended for his two surgical follow-up visits and therefore his care has been put back to his GP.

Teaching the Adult Stoma Patient

Teaching stoma care to the new patient entails an assessment of the patient's readiness to learn and his or her cognitive and psychomotor abilities to understand strategies for appliance changing. The life-changing effect of stoma formation, whether the stoma is to be temporary or permanent, leaves the patient facing an altered body image and self-concept. The patient must learn new ways of caring for him- or herself that are different from the expected 'norm'. Good basic teaching principles combined with encouragement to empower the patient towards self-care will ensure that there is effective incorporation of the cognitive and psychomotor skills needed to manage a new way of life.

The patient's expectations of the teacher, in this instance the nurse, will be that they are knowledgeable, competent and able to provide the care and information needed along the path of recovery. The nurse, for her part, will expect the patient to be willing to learn and that the patient can make the necessary changes to his or her personal care and lifestyle (O'Shea, 2001).

Redman (1988) describes three components to learning: psychomotor, cognitive and affective learning. Although cognitive learning is equated with being literate, in patients who are unable to read and write through lack of education, as opposed to disability, cognitive learning can still be achieved. When teaching a patient, the nurse should use the language with which the patient is familiar, pausing frequently to ensure that the patient is not being confused by medical jargon. Once the patient has understood the essential information related to care of the stoma, he or she is able to move towards self-care.

Understanding a patient's attitudes and values, their affective learning, often starts when the patient first sees the stoma and the response to this stage may define how he or she will behave in the care of the stoma. Attitudes to the physical change in the body and change in the body image picture play a large part in the affective learning of the care of the stoma. The patient has to cope not only with his or her own body change, but also with the attitudes of partner, children, family, relatives, friends and work colleagues. The strong prohibitions on the uncontrolled passage of faeces and urine in western societies, as suggested by Littlewood and Holden (1991), may be a result of the value placed on a post-Cartesian self compared with the socially contextual and reverential notion of the self in non-literate societies. Dirt has been defined as matter out of place, and this implies that there is a set of ordered relations and a contravention of that order. The underlying feeling is that a system of cultural values habitually expressed in a certain arrangement has been violated. Often, individuals who undergo stoma surgery feel stigmatized, a term used by the Greeks to refer to bodily signs indicating something unusual about the person and used in modern medicine to refer to bodily signs of physical disorder (Black, 2000). Overcoming negative feelings about the stoma takes far more time in the new patient and accounts for cognitive learning being quicker than affective learning.

For the patient with a new stoma, learning to care for him- or herself requires a new skill of psychomotor learning. For many new stoma patients this area of learning is accomplished quickly between a few days after surgery and before the patient leaves hospital. The patient often has a fear of what he or she may see when the appliance is removed and this anxiety can be alleviated when the patient has an awareness of what appliance changing entails. The first stage is to understand what equipment is necessary for the patient to form the necessary mental picture of what he or she is going to be doing. The second stage is to understand that the patient is ready by the patient going to the bathroom with the required equipment for an appliance change. Third, the patient undertakes a guided response in changing the appliance, being allowed to take their time in an undisturbed atmosphere. The fourth stage enables the patient to change the appliance while being quietly supervised and, finally, the fifth stage empowers the patient to reach full self-care and go the bathroom as and when necessary to change his or her appliance and to transfer learning from hospital to home; this shows the essential knowledge that is required for successful appliance changing. The first box shows the knowledge needed for successful appliance changing.

In teaching the process of self-care to the stoma patient, the nurse must use assessment, diagnosis, planning, implementation and evaluation, and understand the patient's needs and expectations. During the patient's stay in hospital, he or she has had to take on a lot of new and confusing information about the disease that has caused surgery and a stoma to be raised. Often, in the case of diverticulitis, surgery has been done as an emergency, no preoperative preparation has taken place and the next thing that the patient knows is that he or she has woken up with a stoma. Often the patient can feel so overwhelmed by what has happened in the last hours that his or her attention wanes when different members of the multidisciplinary team all approach at different times with information. It also has to be remembered that patients learn in different ways and use many strategies to cope with learning new ways of caring for themselves with a stoma, and attention span and motivation will occur in periodic plateaux. All of these strategies of learning will help the nurse to understand that stoma instruction cannot be completed in one lesson.

Knowledge needed for successful appliance changing

- What type of stoma do I have? What is the output going to be like? Will the function be different to my normal defecation pattern?
- Do I know why I had to have a stoma? Do I know how long I will have a stoma?
- How do I clean the stoma and skin? How often do I have to do the procedure?
- How do I dispose of the appliance?
- How will I receive new appliances?
- Will I need to eat special meals that are different from the rest of the family?
- Will I be able to go back to work?
- What about the other aspects of my life with my partner and family?

Appliances

Today there is a bewildering supply of stoma appliances available on prescription for the GP to prescribe and the patient to try, and yet most GPs will have little knowledge of what to prescribe for the patient with a new stoma. In addition the community nurse may be as confused about what to advise the patient to use if she has not been actively involved in stoma care for some time. Modern stoma appliances are continuously evolving and changing, and an appliance that the community nurse experienced on a patient last year may not be being frequently used the following year. Hospital specialist stoma care nurses are well placed to know what products are available and what is best suited for the patient at the time of discharge (Black, 1987, 1990, 1994, 1995, 1996, 1997). Factors to be considered when deciding on a suitable appliance for a patient are shown in the second box.

Factors to be considered when choosing an appliance

The person choosing the appliance, whether the stoma care nurse, community nurse or carer, should answer the following questions:

- What type of stoma does the patient have?
- What type of output comes from the stoma?
- Does the patient have full control of their faculties such as sight, hearing, mental ability?
- Does the patient have good manual dexterity?
- What is the patient's lifestyle?
- How and where has the stoma been sited?
- Was the stoma a planned or emergency procedure?
- Does the patient have any experience of stoma appliances or is the patient happy to leave it up to the nurse's experience?

Stoma appliances are divided into three types reflecting the output of the stoma. These are:

1. Colostomy: producing a formed to semi-formed stool.
2. Ileostomy: producing effluent that is fluid and never formed.
3. Urostomy: producing urine.

When surgery is undertaken for diverticulitis, be it emergency or planned surgery, the resulting stoma will be a colostomy. Here, appliances for a colostomy are discussed. However, if more information is needed about ileostomy and urostomy and stoma care, further reading can be found in Black (2000).

Colostomy

A colostomy may be formed in the sigmoid colon, descending colon, transverse colon or ascending colon, and the type of output will depend on the location of the colostomy. When a colostomy is situated in the ascending colon or the transverse colon, the faecal output may vary from a fluid output to a semi-formed stool. For these stomas the optimal appliance to use is a drainable appliance such as would be used if the stoma were an ileostomy. Transverse loop colostomies are often positioned in the upper right quadrant of the abdomen and are usually temporary. Often the size of the stoma when in the transverse position is large, often a loop, and causes difficult management problems for the nurse and patient. Finding a suitable appliance that the patient can use may also cause problems. Often this type of stoma is done on the elderly patient who is debilitated and admitted during the early hours of the morning with a bowel obstruction or problem such as diverticular disease. Emergency surgery is necessary as a result of distal bowel obstruction and to resuscitate the patient. Often, in this situation, the stoma is large and elliptical and the normal plan is to return the patient home to recover in order to readmit later for definitive surgery and closure or revision of the stoma. Although the patient may just be well enough to go home he or she often does not make sufficient recovery to return to hospital for further surgery and the patient and community nurse are left trying to cope with a large and difficult stoma, Today, specialist nurses in stoma care encourage surgeons not to undertake stomas such as these unless it is really necessary.

A colostomy placed in the descending or sigmoid colon will have a faecal output that is generally formed and is easier for the patient to cope with. The appliance will be closed at the bottom and there will be a flatus patch at the top of the appliance that also has charcoal in it. This patch allows gas to escape slowly from the appliance while in wear to prevent the appliance ballooning. The charcoal helps to absorb odours. There are also many other products on the market available to patients who worry about the possibility of odour and that it may offend. These can take the form of powders, capsules, drops or suppository-shaped additives. These additives are put into each new, clean appliance on application and react with the faecal content to help absorb some of the odour. Some of these additives also help with odour when the appliance is being changed (Black, 2000).

Patients who have a colostomy often find it difficult to empty and dispose of stoma appliances, at home or when they are away from home. These patients may benefit from a colostomy appliance disposable in the toilet. Although modern colostomy appliances are one use only, they are not toilet flushable; however, now two colostomy appliances are available that can be flushed down the toilet. One can be removed, folded together and flushed down the toilet. This may take several flushes of the cistern and some help with a toilet brush because the appliance has trapped air inside and tends to float. The other appliance looks like a conventional colostomy appliance but possesses an inner lining. When the appliance needs changing, patients can remove the inner liner and flush it down the toilet and dispose of the plastic outer coat in the normal manner.

Appliances for a sigmoid colostomy or Hartmann's procedure, resulting in an end-colostomy for diverticular disease, may be: a one-piece or two-piece appliance, clear or opaque, with or without a soft cover, with an opaque soft cover over a clear bag but with a slit in the cover to allow the patient to site the appliance correctly, with a cut to fit the aperture or a ready-cut sized aperture. Such are the choices for the patient with a colostomy that most patients expect the nurse to guide them to the correct appliance for the first stage of their rehabilitation.

When the nurse has taken into account the needs of the patient in the use of a colostomy appliance, such as manual dexterity, sight and any other potential problems, it may be suitable to use a one-piece appliance if the nurse considers that it may make changing the appliance easier. A one-piece appliance has an integral adhesive skin wafer, which may have a single release paper or be combined with a microporous collar. In hospital the appliance is clear, without a cover, to allow inspection of the stoma and contents whenever necessary by the doctors and nurses. Often patients do not like being able to see the content of the appliance and choose to have an opaque appliance once at home. Many older patients choose to remain with a transparent appliance because it enables them to place the appliance over the stoma correctly. The aperture in hospital will be cut to fit with the nurse helping the patient by using a template. It is not until the patient has been at home for some time after surgery that the stoma settles to its final size after surgery. At this time the patient is able to use ready-cut apertures, which then does away with the need to cut each aperture on each appliance. If the stoma is not circular, the appliances may need to be cut specially and this can be done by the delivery service that the patient uses for supplies or the chemist from which the patient collects his or her supplies (see 'Discharge and community care' below).

A two-piece appliance consists of an adhesive flange that can have a single release paper and/or a microporous collar. The colostomy appliance attaches to the flange either by clipping together or by adhering to the flange, so making the appliance less bulky and easier for the patient to use. Currently, in the UK, the prevalence of use of one-piece appliances is 82% against 18% of patients who use a two-piece appliance (IMS, 2003). Often for patients who undergo emergency surgery without siting of the stoma, as may be the case in emergency surgery for diverticular disease, the stoma may be in an awkward position and a one-piece appliance with a flexible skin wafer may be the appliance of choice to accommodate the badly placed stoma. Many patients who have badly placed stomas or stomas that have become flush with or retracted below the abdominal surface may benefit from using a flange or one-piece appliance that has convexity built into it. Convexity produces an outward curve on the flange when applied to the stoma and has the effect of pushing the stoma out, which helps the output fall into the appliance rather than leaking out under the flange and causing damage to the peristomal skin. Convexity is available for all types of stomas, but if the stoma is sited preoperatively there should not be a need for convexity. It must be used under supervision of the specialist or community nurse because inappropriate use can cause damage to the stoma (Black, 1996).

For the patient who has an end-colostomy after a Hartmann's procedure for diverticular disease, there are possible alternatives to care of the colostomy that do not need an appliance. Unfortunately, many of the patients who have a colostomy for diverticular disease fall into the older age group and may have other age-associated difficulties that would preclude them from using the following alternatives.

First, provided that the patient is confident with his or her stoma management and if the faecal output is formed, the continent ostomy system is a plug that is inserted into the colostomy. The plug is lubricated and seals off the colostomy by adhering to either the skin or a base plate or flange. When the plug, which has the appearance of a large mushroom, is inserted into the colostomy and secured to the skin or base plate, the lubricated stalk expands with body fluid to block the colostomy outlet. Faecal matter goes on forming and comes up behind the cap. On removal of the plug, an appliance can be put on to secure the collection of faecal output or, if the patient is adept, he or she may be able to excrete into the toilet. At each removal of the plug a new plug has to put in. Often this form of management is useful for social situations with the patient returning to a standard appliance at all other times. The plug can remain *in situ* for up to 12 hours. Patient education is needed before commencing to use the plug and this can be obtained from the specialist stoma care nurse.

For some patients with an end-colostomy there is a way of emptying the bowel daily that also alleviates the wearing of a colostomy appliance. This is irrigation. To do this the patient must be motivated and have the uninterrupted use of a bathroom and toilet each day for at least an hour. There are strict criteria and the irrigation method should be taught by a stoma care nurse or other qualified practitioner in the comfort of the patient's own home. A specialized set to irrigate the bowel is needed and a starter set is usually obtained from one of the ostomy companies; any further replacement pieces are available on prescription. The set comprises a 2-litre bag to hold the hypotonic solution (tap water) to wash out the bowel, tubing and a specialized silicone cone to conduct the water into the colostomy, and a special long bag known as a sleeve to conduct the water from the colostomy into the toilet pan. The patient sits on the toilet and applies the long sleeve to the stoma. The sleeve can be a one- or two-piece item. The bottom of the sleeve is put into the toilet pan. The fluid holder bag is hung on a hook above shoulder height when the patient is sitting on the toilet and the tubing and cone attached. The cone is lubricated and placed through the opening in the top of the sleeve into the colostomy. The fluid control is turned on and up to 1500 ml of water is allowed to flow into the stoma quickly. The patient may start to feel distended at this stage. If the patient feels pain the flow of water should be stopped. Once the cone is removed from the colostomy there will be an immediate return of the water, under pressure, from the colostomy down the sleeve into the toilet. After the initial output the bowel will have a quiet period of 10–15 minutes before the next, slower output of faecal matter. If irrigation is done regularly every 24 hours, within 10 days or so the whole procedure can take as little as 30 minutes to do each day. Patients then can wear a stoma cap each day as opposed to wearing a colostomy bag. All the equipment for irrigation is reusable and needs to be replaced on a yearly basis.

Discharge and Community Care

Successful rehabilitation of the stoma patient back to the community that he or she came from is an essential part of the nurse's job, whether it be the ward nurse or the nurse specialist in stoma care in liaison with the ward team, preparing the patient for a new phase of his or her life (Black, 1990). In a study by Pringle et al. (1997) it was suggested that the poor quality of life and stigma that stoma patients felt appeared to be affected by the level of support available to them once they were discharged. As far back as 1987, Rubin and Devlin suggested that the passage from hospital to home was the weak link in the chain of continuing care and support.

Successful rehabilitation of the stoma patient in the community depends on several factors:

- Understanding the type of stoma and whether it is temporary or permanent.
- Understanding which is the correct type of appliance.
- The correct prescription and supply of appliances, whether from the local chemist or via a delivery service.
- Contact numbers for support from the stoma care nurse in the community, the community nurse or the appropriate voluntary organization.

Often the skills that the patient has learnt in hospital in self-care will have to be adapted to the home situation. With the worry of discharge, often much of the practical management in stoma care is forgotten and the worry of perhaps living on one's own or with an ill spouse brings the stark reality of learning to live with a stoma without medical back-up.

Wade (1989), in her study of stoma care nurses and their patients, looked at the formal support for stoma patients in the community, once they have left hospital. Wade found that, in districts where there were stoma care nurses, up to 93% of patients had received a home visit in the 10 weeks after surgery. Only 7% of patients in non-stoma care nurse districts had received a visit at the same stage. Often, in these areas, the contact with a stoma care nurse had been through their spouse actively trying to find some support for the patient. The full impact and the consequences of stoma surgery are often not felt until patients return home and realize that they have to cope on their own. Often the only contact that patient may have will be with his or her GP, almost invariably at the patient's insistence, and the GP may have little knowledge or time to deal with the practical and psychological problems that the stoma patient may encounter.

One of the biggest anxieties of the stoma patient on leaving hospital is how and where to obtain the appliances. On discharge from hospital, the nurse will have given the patient 2 weeks' supply of the correct appliance for their stoma and, if necessary, the nurse can aid the patient by cutting the appliance to the correct size if a ready-cut appliance is not suitable, either because of the shape of the stoma or because the stoma has not shrunk to its final size after surgery. Normally the patient will be given a choice of a delivery service of appliances to the home or to go to their local chemist and collect the supplies. A prescription from the GP will have to be obtained regardless of the type of service that the patient opts to use. If the patient is 60 years or over, male or female, there is no cost for the prescription. If the patient is under 60 years a form will have to be obtained from the post office or the stoma care nurse that allows the patient an exemption from prescription charges.

Accessories

Apart from appliances, accessories can make up a large part of the GP spend on the few stoma patients that he or she may have in the practice. Accessories are as follows:

- deodorants for odour
- pastes for filling cracks and crevices
- skin protectors that are applied before the appliance
- night drainage bags
- adhesive removers
- appliance covers
- belts
- abdominal supports.

As with many of the prescribable accessories that can be used by the stoma patient, if good stoma care is taught, patients do not routinely need accessories to supplement their stoma appliances.

The cost of caring for the stoma patient in the community takes a large proportion of the GP's budget, especially as stoma appliances are low-volume, high-priced goods. Since the formation of primary care trusts (PCTs) there are unified budgets for prescribing hospital and community health services and therefore it is vital that prescribing costs are kept down. Stoma care products are an area that GPs find difficult to assess; they normally rely on the stoma care nurse or discharging nurse on the ward to supply the correct information for the patient's prescription. If a patient just requests stoma bags from a GP it is unlikely that the GP would be able to prescribe the appropriate appliance unless the patient had the full and correct information.

In 1997, stoma goods accounted for 1.3 million prescription items costing £89 000 000 – 2% of prescribing costs in England for that year. After the first prescription for stoma appliances is provided by the GP, the following prescriptions are done on a repeat request programme and the prescription is automatically signed by the GP. In the face of escalating practice costs, GPs start to look at prescribing and search for areas where money can be saved and stoma appliances are often targeted.

Sometimes, accessory products are needed by the patient for short-term or one-time use, but unless the product is removed from the prescription after the need has finished the product will go on being prescribed and the patient will often stockpile the accessory. For GPs the use of prescribing analysis and cost data (PACT) can be a useful tool to audit stoma appliance prescribing within their PCT. Prescribing data are kept by the Prescribing Prescription Authority (PPA) and include the name, cost and number of items dispensed. This information is available at national, health authority and practice levels and can allow the GP to examine a specific therapeutic area such as stoma care. Armed with this information the GP can highlight his or her spend on stoma appliances. It seems that GPs find the large and constantly changing number of stoma products that become available bewildering, and many do not have the expertise to identify the inappropriate or excessive usage of certain products (Majeed, 1998).

If GPs undertook regularly to audit stoma patients in their practice, either in conjunction with their stoma care nurse or by seeing the patient at least once a year to rewrite the patient's prescription and remove appliances or accessory products that are not currently needed, considerable savings could be made within the PCT.

Hidden Problems in Stoma Care

As the proportion of people aged over 65 continues to grow, the proportion of elderly patients with stomas continues to grow (Ebersole and Hess, 1998). Currently, in the UK the average life expectancy is 83 years for men and 87 years for women. Certain areas of the UK, especially on the south coast of England, have high populations of people over the age of 70 years – as high as 27.9%. In 2000, 10.6% of the population was over the age of 80 (Black, 2000). For many of these patients, there are already other long-standing physical problems and cognitive problems which are going to be complicated further by stoma surgery. For those patients needing to learn self-care for their new stoma, individual assessment of the patient's psychological and cognitive function will be needed to assess how teaching strategies can be adapted. Fine and gross impairment in motor skills will complicate package opening, skin cleansing and appliance application. Visual and hearing impairments make it difficult to understand everything that is being said in teaching situations, and alteration of teaching patterns will be needed to cope with these situations. Although older patients may be effective practitioners, they require a longer period of time to learn appliance application and this often entails a longer hospital stay until the patient feels able to cope on discharge home.

Long-term memory is often better than short-term memory in elderly people, so they find it difficult to repeat something that has been shown to them the day before. To help with this it is easier if teaching can be associated with their long-term memory. In instructing the older patient a quiet environment is needed where there will be no continual interference, such as a need by others to use the bathroom, the telephone ringing or bleeps going off. Even if the patient has not admitted to a hearing impairment, the nurse should face the patient during teaching and use straightforward sentences as opposed to medical jargon. Although written information may be given, the patient may be unable to read adequately or not at all. If it has been ascertained before teaching the patient that there is an inability to read, written information on appliance changing can be given in picture form, using pictures put together from the various patient teaching booklets. Those patients with visual acuity problems may manage better with enhanced light or may need sunlight reduced if the room is too bright. For those who are blind the use of tapes and Braille cards helps reinforce teaching.

A fear that many elderly people have is that their spouse may be asked to help with the changing of the appliance and that they will become dependent on another. The family may worry that they will have to have the relative to live with them after discharge from hospital or may be asked to participate in some part of the patient's care. Family support and acceptance of the ostomate are essential for the successful rehabilitation of the patient and his or her discharge back into the community. Usually patients with diverticular disease who have had a stoma are in the older age group (see Chapter 7) and feel that they will find it difficult to continue in their own home, and may express the wish to sell their home and move into a nursing home or sheltered accommodation because they feel that they will not be able cope with a stoma. At this stage patients should be encouraged not to make any wide-ranging decisions until they have had a chance to go home and assess their situation as they begin to recover from surgery.

Often, for some elderly patients admitted as an emergency for surgery for diverticular disease, it may be the first time that they have been into hospital for an extended period of time and had an operation. Some elderly people with diverticular disease will put up with severe pain at home and try not to be admitted to hospital. They may well be debilitated and confused on admission, as well as having pain, and be put in a bed with cotsides next to a stranger. Some will have difficulty in understanding staff from other cultures and some do not understand that there are also male nurses. Faced with the loss of basic bodily functions, disrupted routines and postoperative confusion, elderly patients may feel that they have regressed to childhood and become tearful and aggressive. Elderly people, when informed that a stoma will be needed for their surgery for diverticular disease, will fear that they will have to have a special diet and become worried about the financial implications of this. They should be assured that a special diet is not necessary, but what will be needed is a natural high-fibre diet; it may be necessary to give them written details about what should be eaten. It must be stressed to the patient that, although a list of suitable foods has been written down for them, these are not the only foods that they should eat, but ones that should be included in an all-round healthy diet.

Multicultural Issues

In today's multicultural society there are implications for the nurses and doctors who provide health care for that society. Patients whose culture and beliefs differ from those of the nurse are yet another challenge for the nurse in teaching stoma care.

Planned care must evolve from around the patient's culture and religious beliefs, and it must be determined whether their belief is an orthodox or a secular belief. Awareness and understanding of the multicultural world in which the nurse works and ways of knowing people in different frames of reference is challenging and nurses are beginning to recognize the values and beliefs and health practices of different cultures in order to provide culturally appropriate care that is relevant to the population (Black, 2000).

Nurses are beginning to recognize that, apart from the obvious fact that many patients from ethnic minorities have little or no command of the English language, religion and customs affect the ways in which this group of patients perceive their care. The environmental context in which individuals have been reared may influence health perceptions and health influences. Culture and ethnicity may influence one's physical development and exposure to health-compromising environments and conditions. Culture may also influence the family structure and how individuals respond to health and illness.

For nurses to provide culturally competent care – a complex integration of skills, knowledge and attitudes that cross cultural communication – they must demonstrate respect for others and promote the well-being of the patient. Although a comparatively small number of patients come from ethnic minority groups, a failure by nursing and medical staff to understand their special needs can lead to isolation of individuals on returning to their communities, and indeed they can become outcasts of that society. Smaje (1995) suggests that the contemporary ethnic character of Britain's population was forged in the nineteenth and twentieth centuries, largely as a result of government policies. With this wide ethnic diversity now seen in Britain, it brings to the forefront the need for the NHS to respond appropriately, with cultural and clinical competence, in the provision of care for these groups which until now have occupied a marginal position when it comes to healthcare policy and delivery.

Careful consideration should be given to the influence of cultural differences in stoma management before a teaching plan is designed. Some cultural practices are harmless and can be accepted or ignored, some are harmful to health and the nurse should explain her reservations about the practice. Ultimately the patient and family reserve the right to carry out the practice if, after due explanation, the family feel that it should be continued once at home.

If the patient speaks no English a translator should be used and it is entirely inappropriate to use the ward domestic staff because she or he speaks the same language or dialect. A medical translator should be found who is acceptable to the patient and family. Most hospitals and hospital switchboards keep a list of approved translators from within the hospital or from approved translating services. Occasionally, if the translator is from a non-approved source, the translation of what the patient needs to know may not be what the patient receives. It may be that the translator feels that what the patient has to be told is not suitable and therefore the patient is shocked when unexpected surgery and a stoma are the eventual outcome. It would be impossible for healthcare workers to expect to understand fully all the cultural and religious needs of the ethnic communities with which they come into contact, but they should at least be aware of the ethnic mix of the local community in which they work.

Limited translated leaflets for Pujabi- and Gujurati-speaking patients who are to have a stoma are available from the British Colostomy Association and further information on multicultural aspects in stoma care can be found in Black (2000).

CARING FOR YOUR STOMA: A PATIENT GUIDE

Before changing your appliance make sure everything you need is ready and at hand. You will need:

- A clean appliance with the correct size aperture already cut
- Any accessories that have been recommended
- Disposal bag for rubbish and dirty appliance
- Flannel or dry wipes
- Towel
- Toilet roll
- Scissors if required
- Soap and warm water.

Make sure that you are comfortable in the bathroom and will not be disturbed. Make sure that the bathroom is of the correct heat and if necessary that you have a chair or stool to sit on.

- Secure clothing out of the way. Rather than tucking under the chin, use clothes pegs to hold clothing up.
- Remove old appliance carefully, top to bottom, easing the adhesive away from the skin. It may be useful to stand on some newspaper or plastic if you are worried about spills.
- Wipe any excess faecal matter away with toilet paper, then wash the stoma and area around the stoma with soap and water.
- After cleaning thoroughly, using a mirror if need be to see all areas, dry with a dry wipe or soft towel.
- If any skin protection has been prescribed apply to clean, dry skin and allow to dry for a few seconds. Do not use creams that have not been prescribed.
- Remove the backing paper from the appliance and position over the stoma, if necessary using a mirror to ensure correct placement.

DISPOSING OF THE APPLIANCE

- Cut the colostomy appliance at the bottom and empty contents down the toilet. Hold the appliance at the top either by hand or with a peg and hold under the flush of the toilet. This is adequate to rinse out the appliance.
- Place soiled appliance and dirty wipes in disposal bag and secure, then place in dustbin.
- Wash hands and restock appliance carrier.
- Try to find a routine that suits you best.
- Make sure that you have adequate appliances and do not forget that at times of public holidays you may need to order earlier than you would normally.
- If you have just been discharged from hospital your stoma may still be changing in size; you should measure the stoma weekly with a stoma guide and change the template accordingly.

Chapter 9
Cultural Issues

Diverticular disease of the large bowel in western societies is common and it appears that the prevalence of this disease increases with age (Horner, 1958; Hughes, 1969; Parks, 1968; Sim and Scobie, 1982; Thompson et al., 1982). Much of the population in Europe, North America and Australia may develop the disease and it is often quoted by healthcare professionals that diverticular disease is rare among African peoples; yet Africans adopting a western lifestyle become susceptible to the disease (Keeley, 1958; Burkitt et al., 1985). It was noticeable that war-time Britons and vegetarians whose diet is high in fibre appear to be less susceptible to the disease, therefore reinforcing the view that the disease is one of western civilization resulting from a fibre-deficient diet (Almy and Howell, 1980). In the USA, the minority with complications of the disease (200 000 hospitalizations per annum) cost three quarters of a billion US dollars annually in healthcare bills (US Department of Health, Education and Welfare, 1979).

In a comparison of European and non-European communities, Kyle et al. (1967), researched populations served by main teaching hospitals in Fiji, Singapore, Nigeria and northern Scotland by four surgeons, all of whom were known to each other. In looking at the results of this trial, using admission to hospital as a reflection of the incidence of the disease, it appears that there is very little diverticulitis among Africans, Chinese, Malay and Indians in Singapore. Yet the incidence among Europeans in Fiji and Singapore indicates that they have admission rates for diverticulitis 40 times higher than those of other inhabitants on these islands (Kyle et al., 1967).

There are possible explanations for the difference in admission rates for the Europeans, or those of European derivation, as against the population of Africans, Asians and Melanesians. Racial differences in epidemiological studies are often difficult to separate from cultural, dietary and other extrinsic factors. One factor in the study may be the way the population seek healthcare advice.

Cultural Attitudes

Black (2000) describes explanatory models and semantic networks used by patients and healthcare workers who may have preconceived ideas about patterns of illness and how that illness should be interpreted and treated. Kleinman (1980) describes five core points used to distinguish notions about episodes of sickness and treatment. He describes these as core clinical functions of how systems of medical knowledge and practice enable people:

- culturally to construct illness as a psychosocial experience
- to establish general criteria to guide the health-seeking process and evaluate the treatment approach
- to manage particular illness episodes by communication, labelling and explanation
- to engage in healthy activities and therapeutic interventions, medicine, surgery, healing rituals and counselling
- to manage the therapeutic outcome and appropriate treatments for the condition.

These five care points or notions about sickness and illness have been described by Kleinman as explanatory models. The clinical process is one way for the individual to adapt to certain worrying circumstances, e.g. abdominal surgery and the possibility of the formation of a stoma. The adaptation premise is reflected in Kleinman's choice of words such as managing, coping, guiding, explaining and negotiating alliances (Young, 1982). Malfunctioning of the body and the psychological processes involved become disease, and the psychosocial disruption becomes illness. Apart from surgery, the first stage of healing is a construction of illness from disease to form a coping function. It may be that a constructional reordering of cultural meaning is all that is necessary in the form of therapy to aid the patient's recovery after surgery.

Culturally, often the use of healers is called upon in non-westernized countries, and these healers have an arcane knowledge and are deemed to have great powers. Their principal social function is to diagnose and prescribe ritual actions to overcome illness or form a prognosis; they name and explain and form explanatory models. As all beliefs are culture bound, little sense can be made of them outside the cultural context. They will also change as the society in which they exist changes and as newer beliefs displace, merge or coexist within the society's older beliefs.

The lay explanatory model is put together in response to a particular episode of illness and is not the same as the individual's general beliefs about illness that his or her society may hold. By contrast, the physician's explanatory model is based on scientific logic and deals with a single cause. Doctor and patient, each using his or her own explanatory model, must agree about the interpretation of each model, the individual's subjective view of the illness and the doctor's view of the disease process. Any problems must be resolved by negotiation so that the patient will comply with the prescribed treatment.

Metaphors of ill health, especially when they are attached to serious conditions relating to the bowel, carry with them a range of associations that can affect how sufferers perceive their condition and how people behave towards them. Bowel movement, for example, is associated with an opening up, allowing entry into the body, the opposite of closing. Assorted words used here are 'empty', 'loosen up', 'unblock', and these suggest that a change has taken place in the internal space of the gut. Having one's bowels emptied is a physical reality associated with internal space and purity – the person is made clean because the bowels are empty. This is often seen when bowel preparation is given before bowel surgery so that the doctor may have unimpeded access to the organ. It is often said that people 'locate' themselves in their bowels and it is considered that the removal of the contents of the bowel may be parallel to removal of self, becoming void, nothing. The very basic personal and private functioning of the individual's bowels in the public domain is also a defining boundary. Young (1982) has suggested that these metaphors of illness emerge at a time when under- standing is experiential and empirical. Terminology, folklore and metaphor are all used in semantic networks and make pathways linking the symbolic to the effective, and language links vocal experience to disease (Turner, 1967).

Linguistically, the 'bowels' are used by the British to express collective anger. British people are thought not to pay much attention to their bodies, yet have a fixation about their bowels. To have a bowel action every day is for many a necessity and the bowel is thought to be the cesspool of the unemptied colon. Constipation is defined by many British people as not having their bowels open every day, a belief that goes back to earlier days when it was thought that the intestinal contents putrefy, forming toxins, leading to poisoning of the body. Black (1992), in a small qualitative study, found that people in the research sample often considered that the individual's bowel problem was caused by the contents becoming putrefied, leading to poisoning of the body, as in diverticulitis. Illness episode schedules showed the use of semantic networks and explanatory models in descriptions of why the individual had become ill. One patient considered that his illness was retribution for abuse of his body by eating the wrong food, whereas some thought toxins in the air to be the cause. An Asian patient considered that he had let his inner self go, and the disease had then attacked. If a framework is to be developed to understand the relationship between disease and language, it is important that the disease is observed as a sociohistorical and cultural phenomenon. Into this network the doctor intervenes diagnostically and therapeutically (Good, 1977) and to build a structural theory in body imagery it is important that semantic networks are researched (see Chapter 8).

When epidemiological studies are undertaken, it is often difficult for biomedical researchers to separate cultural, racial, dietary and other factors to give a true picture of what may be causing certain diseases. Chang (1965) noted that the incidence of diverticulitis in the Japanese population in Hawaii was lower than in Europeans in Hawaii. However, in native Hawaiians, who make up 16% of the population, there were only 2% of cases with diverticulitis. Kim (1964) stated that diverticulitis was rarely found in Koreans, and the authors of the previously discussed research (Kyle et al., 1967) found that their enquiries in northern Japan, the Punjab, Nepal and southern Iran concluded that diverticulitis was rarely, if ever, seen in these communities. If, in the preceding group of countries, the populations are considered to be as racially different from each other as they are from Europeans, perhaps the racial factor in epidemiology needs to be investigated.

In Scandinavia, diverticulosis, seen more frequently as the precursor to diverticulitis, is more common in southern Sweden than in its neighbour Finland. It is recognized that Sweden and Finland have good standards of healthcare in western Europe and good standards of living, yet the two countries have different ethnic origins, the Swedish being Nordic and the Finns being from the east Baltic regions (Kohler, 1963).

Diverticular disease in Africa

It is often postulated that diverticular disease is virtually unknown in black Africans who live south of the Sahara in rural environments and who have not changed their traditional high-residue diet (Segal et al., 1977). As many black South Africans began to move from the rural areas to urban industrialized areas around Johannesburg, their social and educational development became more sophisticated than their rural counterparts. When comparing the dietary intake of the two groups of black South Africans, the rural and urbanized, a major difference is seen in fibre intake. The rural diet consists mainly of maize, millet and wheat products, plus beans, dried peas, ground nuts, vegetables and fruit. Milk and meat are not often included in the diet. As a result of the social and educational upward movement of the urbanized black South African who may be in domestic employment, the diet becomes very similar to that consumed by western populations with low fibre and low residue and high in sugar.

In the small study undertaken by Segal et al. (1977) the cohort came from urbanized black south Africans who regularly consumed a high refined carbohydrate diet. The staple diet of the rural black South African, which is maize, was not eaten by the cohort; fruit was rare and vegetables were eaten only once a week. Meat was part of the diet on a daily basis. Radiological studies in the form of barium enemas showed that six patients had isolated diverticula, whereas 10 demonstrated multi-diverticula as would be seen in patients from western countries.

The postulated aetiological relationship put forward in the much quoted Painter and Burkitt paper (1975) appears to be confirmation that a change in dietary fibre intake has a bearing on the association of fibre and diverticular disease. In the South African study the cohort are the first generation who have given up traditional foods and changed from a high to low residue diet.

In studying the Bantu, an African tribe who solely use the healthcare facilities of the Baragwanath Hospital in Johannesburg, Keeley (1958) reviewed the postmortem examinations of 2367 patients between the years 1954 and 1956 for diverticulosis. Of this group 789 were over 45 years of age. The incidence was just one case. Clinically and radiologically, diverticulitis had been identified only once. A. Solomon, in a personal communication in 1969 to Painter and Burkitt (1975), had, in a 3-year period to 1971, reported six cases of diverticula in 1000 consecutive barium enemas.

In Kampala, only two cases of diverticula were identified by Davies (quoted in Trowell, 1960) from 4000 postmortem examinations in 15 years. In other areas of Africa, Nairobi, Congo, Durban and Ghana over periods of surgical experience ranging from 8 to 16 years, diverticula were identified on fewer than 10 occasions (F. Badoe, 1969; D. Chapman, 1969; M.S.R. Hutt, 1970; A. Jain, 1970; J.R. Miller, 1970; A.L. Templeton, 1970 – cited in Painter and Burkitt, 1975). It could be suggested that some facilities in African hospitals are not as good as they are at major hospitals and therefore the incidence of diverticula could easily be missed, but this was unlikely at major hospitals where there was plenty of experience, especially in the pathology department. These results contrast sharply with the results of 221 barium enemas on white South Africans, in whom 20.8% were shown to have diverticula (Segal et al., 1977).

The conclusions of this study appear to be that the ongoing urbanization of the black South African has seen the accompaniment of diverticular disease which had been virtually unknown in this population. The recognition of any disease pattern will depend on the researcher and awareness of the occurrence in a specified population. Consideration must be given to the dietary intake and any other habits such as socioeconomic conditions, geographical origin, and local or tribal customs.

Diverticular disease in Singapore

Diverticular disease is common in the west but rare in the east (Painter and Burkitt, 1969). The importance of high fibre has been discussed and is considered important in helping to prevent this condition. In the consumption of a low-fibre diet, not only is there the risk of developing diverticular disease, but there is also the possibility of a low-fibre diet being the precursor to appendicitis and colorectal cancer.

Appendicitis and colorectal cancer are common in Singapore and colorectal cancer is rising to become the main malignant neoplasm in the twenty-first century. Early studies in Singapore show that clinically diagnosed diverticular disease is relatively rare (Kyle et al., 1967).

Before 1986, 1014 consecutive large bowels from people aged 14 and over were examined postmortem. The whole of the bowel from anus to caecum was opened and cleaned and examined for diverticula. All positive cases were confirmed histologically. Ethnic grouping of the patients was into the three main areas of Chinese, Indian and Malay. It was noted that Chinese men had a larger proportion of diverticular disease (24%) than Malay (11.7%) or Indian (14.3%) men (Lee, 1986).

Right-sided diverticulosis was seen as the predominant pattern in all the postmortem age groups and was particularly prevalent before 40 years of age. This contrasts with findings in a western population of diverticulosis occurring predominantly on the left-side colon in the sigmoid area (Lee, 1986).

Further radiological investigation, done by Chia et al. (1991) using barium enemas as diagnosis, reviewed 524 studies. This study produced a 20% prevalence rate that is equal to western countries such as Sweden and the USA, and is higher than nearby Asian communities such as Thailand, Korea and Hong Kong. Again in Singapore, using a radiological medium, the feature of right-sided diverticulosis was demonstrated.

Studies from developing countries show that diverticular disease is uncommon and some communities will show a different anatomical variation as seen here. However, as a community becomes more developed and adopts a diet low in fibre, and high in saturated fat and meat, diverticular disease will be seen more often (Ellis, 1970; Painter and Burkitt, 1971). Over the last 20 years Singapore has progressed economically from being a developing country to the second richest in Asia and the twentieth in the whole world. With this has come the adoption of a low-fibre, refined diet as seen in the western world.

Chia et al. (1991), Vajrabukka et al. (1980) and Lee (1986) suggest that their data show that a predominantly Oriental population appear to develop right-sided diverticular disease, whereas a European population develop left-sided diverticulosis. Therefore, the anatomical site for diverticular disease is racial and genetic, although the prevalence is environmental and related to diet and low fibre. (See Table 9.1.)

Table 9.1 Diverticular disease in the Far East

Source	Study	Incidence (%)	No.	Right sided (%)
Singapore Lee (1986)	PM	19.0	1014	66.3
Japan Sugihara et al. (1984)	Barium	13.3	1839	68.6
Hong Kong Coode et al. (1985)	PM	5.0	200	70.0
Thailand Vajrabukka et al. (1980)	Barium	4.2	289	66.7
Korea Munakata et al. (1982)	Barium	0.3	3239	70.0

Adapted from Chia et al. (1991).

Diverticular disease in New Zealand

In investigating colorectal disorders at Wellington Hospital in New Zealand, Sim and Scobie (1982) analysed 1118 air contrast enemas and found 395 with diverticular disease. Complicated diverticular disease was rare although an analysis of specific symptoms with uncomplicated diverticular disease, such as pain, bowel habit and bleeding, was no different from patients with negative barium enemas.

In 1975, air contrast barium enemas became routine, allowing increased accuracy compared with a standard barium enema. Diverticular disease increased with age from 4% in the 30s rising to 66% in the 90s. Diverticular disease affected the sigmoid colon severely in 13 patients, moderately in 303 patients and to a minor degree in 70 patients.

Gross disease was found in 13 patients involving most of the colon. Atypical sites were found in eight patients, four in the ascending colon, three in the splenic flexure and one in the hepatic flexure. Of the complicated diverticular disease, one suggested an involvement of a pelvic colorectal cancer, one with a vesicolic fistula demonstrating gas in the bladder, one with stenosis, one perforated and two with masses.

The incidence of diverticular disease in New Zealand concurs with postmortem findings in Australia, the UK and France (Debray et al., 1961; Parks, 1968; Hughes, 1969). Although large bowel disease such as cancer, polyps, inflammatory bowel disease and diverticular disease are noted to be diseases of the western world resulting from fibre deficiency, there has been no in-depth analysis in New Zealand, although the paper by Sim and Scobie (1982) has begun to address these issues.

Diverticular disease in Scandinavia

In radiological contrasts undertaken by Kohler (1963) on a Finnish and southern Swedish population, he found that the contrast enema rarely showed diverticular disease in the Finnish population, yet using the same radiological medium diverticular disease appears to be more common among the southern Swedish population. Although diverticular disease can be demonstrated by radiological studies with barium enemas and by double contrast, much of the statistical evidence is dominated by the UK and America.

As far back as 1925 there were studies indicating that there may be a racial difference that predisposes to diverticular disease and Larimore (1925) suggests that it is higher among the white than the black population. Hilden (1933) suggested that European racial variations were a contributing factor to the disease. The Nordic race, from which the Swedes descend, is a different race from the one from which the Finnish people descend. The Finnish people descend from the east Baltic race. Diverticulosis was seen in 5.2% of 3125 Finnish patients, whereas in the Swedish group diverticulosis was seen in 15.8% of 3563 patients. In both groups the incidence increased with age. In the Swedish series the diverticulosis was seen in the sigmoid colon, but in the Finnish series diverticulosis was seen in other segments of the colon. Eighty-six per cent of diverticulosis cases in Swedish patients occurred in the sigmoid or descending areas whereas only 66% occurred in the same bowel area in the Finnish patients. The Swedish figures correlate to the UK and US statistics.

A comparison on the same level as the Scandinavian study was undertaken in Utah, USA by Smith and Christensen in 1959, and the results were similar to the Swedish arm of Kohler's study (1963).

Although the incidence of diverticulosis in the colon appears to be three times higher in southern Sweden than in southern Finland, it is difficult to ascertain the reasons why. Although complex and not defined precisely, racial and genetic differences may be inherent, along with diet, mobility, socioeconomic factors and general way of life.

Diverticular disease in the Japanese in Hawaii

The Japanese are the second most numerous population to reside in Hawaii and offer the researcher a wider population of sex, age and long-term residence. The class level of the Japanese in Hawaiian society is that of a middle-class society.

Diverticulitis in Hawaiian Japanese differs from that found in other races in Hawaii and occurs most often on the right side in the ascending colon (Stemmermann, 1970). This correlates with the incidence of right-sided diverticulitis previously discussed, seen in the population from far eastern countries. Chang (1965) demonstrated that 62.3% of 85 patients admitted to three hospitals in Honolulu were Japanese and the average age of patients with right-sided diverticulitis is about 20 years younger than those who experience diverticulitis on the left-sided colon.

Although some disease patterns in the Japanese in Hawaii have not seen any changes, less common diseases such as right-sided diverticulitis seem to be increasing.

Diverticular disease in Greece

An epidemiological study looking at biosocial factors and diet in Athens was undertaken by Manousos et al. (1985) using the dietary availability that is known in Greece, which enables an epidemiological study to be satisfactorily undertaken. A hundred cases of diverticulosis confirmed by barium enema radiological studies were hospitalized in Athens. These were consecutive cases who had been diagnosed for the first time with diverticulosis. Dietary histories were obtained and also socioeconomic and demographic details.

Specifically, in this study, the dietary intake was a prime factor and patients were asked about their food consumption. Eighty food items and beverages were categorized and patients were asked about the consumption of these items in categories of daily, weekly and monthly consumption. The food items were grouped and individualized as described by Davidson and Passmore (1979). The frequency and consumption of food were itemized in terms of the number of times per month that the food was consumed. Assignment values were given to foods eaten daily, twice a week, once a week, once a month and not often at all. Of the 100 cases with diverticulosis 66 were aged 60 years or more and lived in Athens or another urban area. This population has a substantial dietary variability and the outcome of the study supports the theory that diet is of importance in diverticular disease.

A fibre increase does not necessarily mean that there will be a reduction in the risk of symptomatic diverticulosis because the disease is not just a fibre-deficient disease. There is a role played by lamb and beef and dairy products in possibly influencing the development of symptomatic diverticular disease. Therefore, the involvement of several dietary factors in the aetiology of diverticular disease may help to explain why vegetarians have a lower asymptomatic prevalence of diverticulosis. The findings of the Athens study are that people who attend hospital with abdominal complaints and undergo radiological tests, such as barium enema, which show diverticulosis, appear to have dietary habits with a considerable difference from those attending hospital for orthopaedic problems and used as a control group. In looking for the cause of a common western disease, case-control studies in a population with varied dietary habits, homogeneous make-up and a low incidence of western disease should be of value (Heaton, 1985).

Chapter 10
Gender and Age in Diverticular Disease

Although literature subscribes to the view that Littre, in 1732, was the first to mention diverticular disease, his description of 'diverticular hernia' was not explained. The first description is attributed to Sommering in his translation into German of *Baillie's Morbid Anatomy* in 1794 (Oschner and Bargen, 1935).

In 1968, Parks reported on the natural history of diverticular disease and found that women were more likely than men to be affected with up to 60% of patients being women. Since 1968, little work has been done to look at the difference in gender in diverticular disease. Other reported studies that have addressed selected complications of diverticular disease have made mention of gender, but there is no single study that is comprehensive and comes from an individual institution investigating all diverticular complications. In 2002, McConnell et al. presented a paper at the Tripartite Colorectal Meeting in Melbourne, Australia documenting their study of the population-based incidence of complicated diverticular disease of the sigmoid colon based on gender and age (McConnell et al., 2003). For a decade, between January 1988 and January 1998, a retrospective review was undertaken of all surgical patients admitted with proven diverticular disease that required surgery. Between January 1999 and December 1999 all patients who underwent flexible sigmoidoscopy were examined to determine the incidence of diverticular disease in the population. Patients were divided into categories of gender and age.

In the decade that was retrospectively examined for patients requiring surgical treatment, 934 were admitted to the department of Colorectal and General Surgery in the Mayo Clinic, Rochester, USA; 443 were male and 491 were female, with an average age of 64 years. Women appeared to present 5 years later than their male counterparts. In the flexible sigmoidoscopy group 10 037 operations were performed within the year period, with 5101 men and 4936 women of average age 57.58 years. Tables 10.1–10.3 show the complications and comparisons of age and gender.

Table 10.1 Comparisons of complications of diverticular disease (DD) between sexes

Complications	Male	Female	Total
Bleeding	34	15	49
Chronic/recurrent DD	148	181	329
Obstruction	25	36	61
Fistula	75	73	148
Perforation	82	88	170
Abscess	37	42	79
Stricture	21	38	59
Acute DD	21	18	39
Total	443	491	934

From McConnell et al. (2003).

Table 10.2 Comparisons of complications of diverticular disease (DD) between age groups

Complications	< 50 years	> 50 years
Bleeding	2	47
Chronic/recurrent DD	64	265
Obstruction	4	57
Fistula	11	137
Perforation	20	150
Abscess	21	58
Stricture	3	56
Acute DD	8	31
Total	133	801

From McConnell et al. (2003).

Table 10.3 Comparisons of complications of diverticular disease (DD) by age and sex

Complications	Men < 50 years	Women < 50 years	Men > 50 years	Women > 50 years
Bleeding	2	0	32	15
Chronic/recurrent DD	42	22	106	159
Obstruction	3	1	22	35
Fistula	10	1	65	72
Perforation	6	14	76	74
Abscess	9	12	28	30
Stricture	3	0	18	38
Acute DD	6	2	15	16
Total	81	52	362	439

From McConnell et al. (2003).

Colonic diverticular disease is common in elderly people, with an increase in incidence as high as 30% in the eighth decade (McConnell et al., 2003) and up to 50% in the ninth decade (Biondo et al., 2002). The early studies show a male preponderance but recent studies still indicate a slight female preponderance, as Parks originally reported in 1968. In the Mayo Clinic review of complicated diverticular disease, males made up most patients aged below 40 years. Although diverticular bleeding that requires surgical intervention is considered to be a disease of elderly people, the population in the Mayo study found 31% of its patients to be younger than 70 years; of those 73% were male.

In looking at complications of diverticular disease, stricture of the sigmoid colon affects 5-25% of patients. Women older than 50 years were found to be twice as likely to develop a stricture that would require surgical intervention. Stricture of the sigmoid colon was found to be more common in the older patient with only 55 being younger than 50 years.

Obstruction of the colon complicating diverticular disease is rare with only a 10% incidence in all large bowel obstructions. Complete obstruction would occur when there is an acute abscess over a chronic stricture. Partial obstruction is more likely to occur when there is oedema and spasm or inflammatory changes. In the Mayo Clinic review no gender differences were reported in this area, with only 6.5% presenting before the age of 50 years and 63% older than 70 years.

The common complication of diverticular disease is diverticulitis, which may be acute or chronic. Nearly 80% of patients with acute diverticulitis recover sufficiently with medical treatment. Recurrent diverticulitis is thought to occur in as many as 7-35% of all patients irrespective of age and gender (Horgan et al., 2001). In patients aged under 40 years there are mixed reports of gender differences, notably with a preponderance of males (Reisman et al., 1999). In the Mayo Clinic study, of patients over 50 years, chronic diverticulitis presented in 111 men and 165 women.

Fistulae may complicate diverticular disease and are common; as many as 20% of patients may require surgery. In a study by Woods et al. (1988) it was found that, of 84 patients with colovesicular fistulae associated with diverticular disease, there was a 2:1 male preponderance. Women may be prevented from colovesicular fistula formation if they have a uterus. In the Mayo Study group 148 patients had colovesicular fistulae associated with diverticular disease and requiring surgery; 73 patients were female and 75 male. Of the female cohort 51% had previously undergone a hysterectomy; 7.4% of patients in this group were under the age of 50 years and only one was female.

The most worrying aspect of diverticular disease for surgeons is a colonic perforation. Although some perforation may wall off and create an abscess, peritonitis requires an emergency operation. Although there is not much in the literature to correlate age, gender and perforation in diverticular disease, one review reports an average of 44.7 years and another of 60 years (Tudor et al., 1994; Schwesinger et al., 2000). In McConnell et al.'s (2003) review, 170 patients of the cohort required surgical intervention as a result of perforation, with 11.7% of both sexes presenting before the age of 50 years. Women aged below 50 years were more commonly affected than men.

In Lee's (1986) survey in Singapore, 194 cases were found to have diverticular disease, which was evident in the large colon after the second decade; men were more frequently affected than women before the age of 60. Chinese men showed more diverticular disease than Malaysian and Indian men and Chinese men showed a significantly higher rate of diverticular disease than Chinese women. There was no significant difference between the prevalence of diverticular disease in Chinese and Indian women. In this survey there was far more right colon involvement (discussed in Chapter 9) with the disease affecting the caecum and ascending colon. In the three major ethnic groups in Singapore, this pattern was observed and occurred in both Singapore-born and foreign-born Singaporeans.

Diverticular disease starts to appear as early as the second decade in Singaporeans and in men the prevalence and rise were seen to be early and rapid, reaching a peak between the fifth and sixth decades, then rapidly dropping off. In women, the age prevalence of diverticular disease was low before the fifth decade, but rose sharply in the sixth decade, peaking in the eighth decade and showing only a small decline thereafter, compared with the sharp drop in later life experienced by men.

Although the relationship between physical activity and diverticular disease has not been directly studied, Aldoori et al. (1995) looked at a cohort of American men as a prospective study. They were aged between 40 and 75 years and diagnosed as free of diverticular disease before 1988. During the prospective study over 4 years, 382 new cases of symptomatic diverticular disease were recorded. Within the USA symptomatic diverticular disease accounts for 200 000 hospital admissions per year. Questionnaires based on self-report physical activity were given and the participants had to report on the average time per week spent at the identified activities, which were graded as moderate or vigorous. Dietary intake, as another variable, was used in a semi-quantitative questionnaire form. In follow-up questionnaires to the cohort every 2 years, participants were asked about diverticular disease during the previous 2 years. Response rates remained high and in 1992 were

94% at the time of analysis. The prospective data suggested that males who undertook physical activity and vigorous activity had a reduced risk of diverticular disease. Men who were more likely to have a higher risk of diverticular disease were those who took little physical activity and also had a dietary intake with low fibre.

As has been previously discussed, diverticulosis is common in elderly people, with the incidence reaching 50% in the ninth decade. The frequent reason for admission to hospital is the acute complication of diverticular disease. Among surgeons there is agreement that fistula, stenosis and haemorrhage in diverticular disease necessitate surgery, but there still is controversy about the treatment of young patients and their management of diverticulitis. It has been suggested that elective resection should be considered in young patients, i.e. under 50 years of age, when an acute infective episode is successfully managed conservatively, and that surgery should be considered because of the recurrent nature of diverticulitis and the possible complications (Konvolinka, 1994; Anderson et al., 1997). However, other authors report that, in patients aged under 40 years, diverticulitis does not have an aggressive nature (Ambrosetti et al., 1994; Spivak et al., 1997).

A study by Biondo et al. (2002) looked at the outcomes and management of diverticulitis in young patients and reported on the management, virulence and outcomes of acute diverticulitis with respect to age. In this study 22% of patients were first-time admissions under the age of 50 years. Ambrosetti et al. (1994) reported that patients younger than 50 years were more likely to have recurrences after conservative treatment, although older patients were more likely to require surgical intervention at first hospital admission. Biondo et al. (2002) found among his cohort that only 1 of 12 patients aged under 50 and 3 of 40 patients aged over 50 needed emergency surgery at the second attack of diverticulitis. However, in this study there was no specific evidence about the aggressive nature of diverticular disease in the young. The severity of peritonitis, as measured by the Hinchey classification, did not alter in either age group. Most patients in both age groups did not require surgery if their condition had responded to medical treatment after the first attack, leading the study's authors to believe that diverticular disease in young patients behaves no differently to the way it behaves in older patients and therefore that it should be managed with the same protocols.

Morbidity and Mortality

The surgical management of left-sided colon emergencies such as diverticular disease and colorectal cancer is moving towards a single surgical procedure but patient selection for a single or staged procedure appears to remain controversial. The choice of operative procedure depends on the patient's health and a single-stage operation is preferable and often achievable even in elderly people with peritonitis, as a result of the advances in intensive care medicine and the management of peritoneal sepsis. Improvement in morbidity, mortality and stoma formation rates is enhanced by the grade of surgeon operating.

In a retrospective study covering 10 years by Zorcolo et al. (2003), 336 patients in a large UK hospital, who presented with an acute abdomen, underwent surgery for left-sided diverticular disease or colorectal cancer without bowel preparation. Patients were operated on by surgeons whose major interest was either colorectal surgery or upper gastrointestinal conditions. Patients were assigned to a particular surgeon by chance, although the colorectal surgeons tended to diagnose and treat more cases.

Of the 336 patients, 65.8% were operated on by the colorectal surgeons and 34.2% by the upper gastrointestinal team. Complicated diverticular disease was present in 58.6% of patients; 193 patients were operated on within 24 hours of admission and the remainder were operated on within 48 hours. Within the whole cohort consultants were present in 197 of the cases, operating in 115 cases and assisting in 82 cases. Registrars were unsupervised in 139 cases. Of the 336 cases, primary anastomosis was made in 184 cases and 15 had a defunctioning stoma. More patients with colorectal cancer had a primary anastomosis compared with those with diverticular disease. Primary anastomosis frequency was indicated by the experience of the operator, with consultants achieving 69.9% and trainees 47%. In patients with diverticular disease the figures were more marked, with consultants achieving 72.7% and trainees 29.8% for a primary anastomosis. In patients who had diverticular disease complicated by peritonitis, a one-stage operation was performed by colorectal surgeons in 37.7% as against 11.5% by non-colorectal surgeons (Zorcolo et al., 2003).

There is an obvious advantage in a one-stage procedure even if sepsis is present, provided that the patient is appropriately selected. Primary anastomosis excludes the high complication rate of reversing a Hartmann's procedure and closing a colostomy. The data from this study suggest that colorectal emergencies have a better outcome if managed by specialist surgeons, reducing stoma rates and complication rates, and with lower mortality rates.

Chapter 11
Food Management in Diverticular Disease

In this chapter we look at the emotive subject of 'diet' in diverticular disease. In changing the terminology to 'food management', this chapter explores the myths and mysteries of the types of food that can and cannot be eaten by a patient with diverticular disease and whether food management can help control it.

As has been discussed in earlier chapters, diverticular disease is a common disorder in the western world affecting between 30% and 50% of the population aged over 60 years (Manousos et al., 1967; Burkitt et al., 1985). Although as many as 6500 patients a year are admitted to hospital for treatment of diverticulitis (Kyle et al., 1967), there are many more attending hospital outpatient departments for investigation of diverticular disease, who will not need surgical intervention. Once diagnosis is confirmed and if surgery is not indicated, there appears to be little left for the doctor to offer the patient to help with the disease. Often doctors call diverticulitis the 'cinderella disease' because there is nothing specific to do for the patient who has an expectation of 'cure' once the investigations are completed. Invariably patients are told that they must follow a 'diet' high in fibre, which will help them. But will 'diet' or food management help patients with diverticulitis? In concentrating on general bowel health, Hill (1999) suggested that fibre therapy should be based on clinical evidence, with the emphasis on the 'prescription' of a specific subtype of dietary fibre for a specific disease. Yet lack of agreement on fundamental issues in the dietary fibre story make it a difficult task when health professionals are giving advice and the current dietary guidelines need to be translated into foods that people can eat in their normal day-to-day living.

Fibre in the Diet

Lack of fibre or a decrease in dietary fibre has been the leading theory in the aetiology of diverticular disease since 1971. Studies undertaken by Painter

90

and Burkitt (1971), using geographical and historical research, have continually received support for this hypothesis. Studies undertaken with case-controls by Brodribb and Humphreys (1976) suggested that patients with diverticular disease had low dietary intakes of crude fibre, but this is not an indicator of overall dietary fibre intake. Gear et al. (1979) and Berry et al. (1984) undertook studies on rats and found that they develop more and more diverticula when they are given less and less bran in their diet. Yet vegetarians have been shown to have less than half the expected prevalence of asymptomatic diverticulosis, which results only partly from their higher fibre intake (Gear et al., 1979).

Although diverticular disease of the colon is viewed as a disease of western civilization and ascribed to inadequate dietary fibre intake, there is a strong clinical impression by the medical profession that increased dietary fibre intake will relieve the symptoms of diverticular disease (Ornstein et al., 1981). In a controlled clinical study, 58 patients with uncomplicated diverticular disease of the colon ingested a bran crispbread, an ispaghula drink (*Psyllium*) and a placebo for 4 months each in a randomized, cross-over, double-masked, controlled trial. Subjective assessments were made monthly using a self-administered questionnaire. Objective studies were made by examination of a 7-day stool collection from each patient at the end of each treatment period. Using a pain and lower bowel symptom score, which included incomplete sensation of emptying the bowel, straining, stool consistency, aperients taken and nausea, and a total symptom score, which included nausea, belching, dyspepsia, vomiting and abdominal distension, it appeared that supplementation with fibre was of no benefit. Benefit from fibre was found for those with constipation while undertaking this regimen. Both regimens of fibre produced the expected changes in stool consistency, weight and frequency of defecation. This trial tested the usual therapeutic dose of bran and ispaghula supplements, which is equivalent to two tablespoons of natural bran, and increased the patients' intake by 50-70%, as opposed to the large quantities of bran used in studies by Painter and Burkitt (1971), Plumley and Francis (1973), Taylor and Duthie (1976) and Brodribb and Humphreys (1976). The conclusion of the above trial showed no difference among the three regimens, although it confirmed that dietary fibre has a well-known and considerable effect on constipation, with ispaghula being better than bran. It was felt that the placebo supplement of 2-3 g dietary fibre in the controlled clinical trial could relieve symptoms while producing fewer objective changes than either bran or ispaghula. The conclusion reached was that, unless the patient's symptoms were those of constipation, dietary fibre supplements are unnecessary in the long-term management of uncomplicated diverticular disease of the colon (Ornstein et al., 1981).

However, the most well-known substantiated theory on the aetiology of diverticular disease is the lack of dietary cereal fibre – a hypothesis put forward by Painter and Burkitt (1975). They had observed that diverticular disease was rarely seen in African countries where dietary fibre intake was high, yet in western countries, where there was a higher incidence of the disease and a lower intake of dietary fibre, they felt that the refining of flour and cereals was the prime cause of diverticulosis. Although this can be confirmed by epidemiological studies, animal experiments and fibre replacement trials (Garry, 1971; Gear et al., 1979; Manousos et al., 1985), few studies are available to show how two other dietary intakes may be relevant to diverticular disease. These are the lack of fresh fruit and vegetables and excess red meat (Aldoori et al., 1998), which can increase the risk of symptomatic disease.

In a cohort study of 48 000 male American health professionals (see Chapter 10) it was found that beef consumption doubled the risk of symptomatic disease and lamb consumption almost quadrupled the disease. Therefore, is red meat a contributory factor to the symptomatic increase of diverticular disease? Although this is a difficult question to answer, this hypothesis considers whether the aromatic heterocyclic amines produced by cooking red meat are the chief offenders. It is known that these compounds can induce neoplasia in animal trials for colonic cancer, but whether they produce diverticular inflammation is not yet known.

The limited intake of fruit and fibre in most people's diets may be a contributing factor to diverticular disease. There is a great deal of publicity recently in the media and shops to encourage people to eat at least five portions of fruit and vegetables each day. Much of this publicity is concerned with the findings that this helps to prevent bowel cancer, but it appears that fibre from fruit and vegetables is as important in the aetiology of diverticular disease as the lack of cereal fibre (Manousos et al., 1985).

Many of the clinical studies have concentrated on treating patients with cereal fibre such as bran or isphagula supplements (Plumley and Francis, 1973; Brodribb and Humphreys, 1976) and the physiological evidence shows that bran can reduce the bowel intraluminal pressure. However, as beneficial as this may be, bran does not abolish the patient's symptoms.

Previously, treatment of diverticular disease was with a low-residue diet and this had been accepted without any proof of its therapeutic value, although medical opinion now favours a high-fibre diet as previously discussed. In the study by Brodribb and Humphreys (1976) in the UK, 40 patients who presented over 12 months with symptoms and underwent a barium enema for diverticular disease were studied. After the initial assessment patients were instructed to take three heaped tablespoons of wheat bran daily and to keep to their normal diet. After 6 months the patients were reassessed and a further barium enema carried out. The original films and the 6-month films were compared and the number of diverticula counted.

All the patients tolerated the bran and said that their symptoms had improved. Of the patients, 60% stated that their symptoms were abolished and 28% that their symptoms were relieved. The study concluded that treatment with cereal fibre can provide good symptomatic relief in patients with uncomplicated diverticular disease and can improve colonic function by increasing stool weight. Changes in barium enema appearances after treatment have a limited clinical significance. Although no decrease of diverticula was seen on radiographs it was noted that there had been no increase either.

Fibre, more than any other dietary component, affects human large bowel function, causing an increase in stool output, dilution of colonic contents, a faster transit rate, and changes in the colonic metabolism of minerals, nitrogen and bile acid (Stephen and Cummings, 1980). It is supposed that these changes are caused by the amount of water that undigested fibre holds within its cellular structure (McConnell et al., 1974; Eastwood and Mitchell, 1976). In this study, two fibres were used to demonstrate that the main component of human faeces is bacteria: cabbage fibre, which is extensively broken down and stimulates microbial growth, and wheat fibre, which remains largely undigested and retains water in the gut lumen. Wheat fibre was seen to survive digestion in the bowel and to alter colonic function by holding water and increasing the bulk of the colonic content. Transit time is decreased and less water is absorbed from the lumen. With cabbage fibre, the faeces were better hydrated than with the wheat, perhaps because the increased bacterial mass stimulated faster transit time and there was less water absorbed from the luminal contents by the bowel mucosa. Cabbage fibre influences colonic function through its stimulation of microbial growth, whereas with wheat fibre there is a smaller increase in the bowel bacteria (Cummings and Stephen, 1980). It has been suggested by Burkitt et al. (1972) that colonic disease is more common in people who have small stool outputs and slow transit time, so the control of colonic microflora is important in determining disease susceptibility in individuals. Therefore, the type, amount and digestibility of fibre in the diet will make a considerable contribution to the microflora.

New Terminology and Guidelines for Fibre Intake

Fibre is a complex food fraction and pharmaceutical and food manufacturers are producing new ranges of products, using research data on fibre to produce functional or therapeutic foods that target specific groups of consumers or patients; this can lead to confusion for the nurse or consumer when trying to understand current health education and the benefit from a higher fibre intake in their diet. If the nurse understands the current issues and new terminology surrounding fibre, she or he will be ideally placed to help and guide the patient with diverticular disease.

The term 'dietary fibre' was described by Hipsley (1953) and it refers to the material that is derived from plant cell walls. Burkitt and Trowell (1975) suggested that the large quantities of unrefined plant foods, with their cell walls intact, which rural Africans ate compared with their western counterparts, were the link in bowel disease, and identified the plant cell wall as the protective factor. To identify these components, Trowell et al. (1976) used the original term that Hipsley (1953) coined – 'dietary fibre'. Trowell and his colleagues (1976) proposed a definition of dietary fibre that became acceptable by most as a convenient working definition at that time.

When proposing new definitions of dietary fibre it is important to consider the indigestibility of these materials; the original term was a complex mixture and the component polysaccharides had a range of chemical and physical properties. Certainly, in the late 1970s, researchers did not readily have the availability of isolated cell wall materials to feed to people to study the mechanism of action.

Burkitt's original hypothesis focused on the effects of indigestible fibre in the colon and its effect on faecal bulk and consistency, intraintestinal pressures, diverticular disease, transit times, atonia, and the effect of bacterial metabolism and bowel cancer. Through research it was seen that substantial proportions of all the components of the plant cell wall, with the exception of lignin, which is a non-carbohydrate, were fermented by microflora in the colon.

At a meeting of a European working party, a newer definition of dietary fibre was proposed. Based on non-digestibility, it states that fibre is:

> The part of the oligosaccharides (shorter chain) and polysaccharides, and their hydrophilic derivatives which cannot be decomposed, by human digestive enzymes, to absorbable components in the upper alimentary tract; it includes lignin.
>
> (Bär, 1993)

In 1987 Englyst et al. had redefined the term 'dietary fibre' by introducing the new terminology NSPs or non-starch polysaccharides. NSPs are categorized as carbohydrates and are considered to be an important constituent of healthy nutrition. Although seen as a carbohydrate, NSP is similar to a starch. Although starch in the diet is used for energy, NSP passes into the colon, where it ferments to produce short chain fatty acids; it is then excreted to help form most of the faecal bulk (Sullivan, 2000). In estimating dietary intake of NSP as part of dietary fibre intake, measurements of NSPs can be analysed in the laboratory. This allows an estimation of dietary fibre intake, appropriate food labelling and informed food choice (Department of Health or DoH, 1991). In 1991 the DoH published *Dietary Reference Values for Food, Energy and Nutrients for the United Kingdom* which described the use of dietary reference values. The Englyst (1994) method of measurement is now used in measuring and this supersedes the older method described by Southgate and Durnin (1970). A recommended daily amount of NSP is 18 g for adults, varying between 12 and 24 g. Realistically, however, in the UK the amount of NSP consumed daily is around 11–13 g, of which 40% is cereal and about 50% is vegetable (DoH, 1991).

The most recent figures from the National Food Survey in 1997, conducted by the Ministry of Agriculture, Food and Fisheries (MAFF, 1997), shows an average consumption of 13.8 g NSP in men and women (Table 11.1). This survey is conducted annually from a random sample of 8000 families across the UK who keep a diary for 7 days of all food bought into the home for human consumption, and an account is also kept of the food and drink consumed outside the home.

Table 11.1 Consumption of non-polysaccharides (NSPs) in adults

Source	NSP (g/day)
MAFF (1997)	13.8
Emmett et al. (1993)	Males: 15.5–16.4 Females: 14.3–15.3
Bingham et al. (1990)	Males: 11.2 Females: 12.5

From Davies (1999).

If, therefore, it seems that the public are not consuming enough health-promoting fibre in the form of NSPs, which has a valuable effect in the prevention and management of a variety of diseases, including bowel dysfunctions and bowel cancer, are fibre supplements the answer? Bulking agents can enhance the intake of NSPs but consumption in this form is not in line with the recommendations of the COMA (Committee on Medical Aspects of Food Policy) panel. It was from the working groups on the COMA panel that the 1991 DoH paper came. NSPs should be derived from a variety of foods with their make-up consisting of a naturally integrated component rather than supplements or enriched NSP products (DoH, 1991).

Diets and Food Labelling

In pursuing the role of health education, nurses are well placed to help clarify the issues that arise about fibre in day-to-day eating. Patients who find that there is so much information to take in at an outpatient appointment with the physician, surgeon or dietician can leave feeling confused and aware that they have not asked the questions that they wanted to, not heard everything that they have been told or felt that they would be wasting time if they asked for things to be repeated. Often nurses are so busy that they do not have time to sit down with patients in the middle of a clinic to go over what they have been told, so they find it easier to resort to a 'diet sheet' and send the patient on his or her way. Is a high-fibre diet sheet the answer? Lambert and Dickerson (1989) surveyed 45 high-fibre diet sheets and found that there were inconsistencies in the importance of consumption of specific fibre-rich foods and that daily meal plans were open to wide interpretation. Eleven recommended bran for everybody, fifteen recommended using it if necessary and nine recommended its use if advised by a doctor and dietician. The use of large quantities of unprocessed bran is not advised because bran renders the minerals zinc, iron and calcium unavailable to the body as a result of its mineral-binding action. If large amounts of fibre are not available for consumption or cannot be consumed, NSPs can be ingested in the form of sterculia, isphagula or methylcellulose, which are bulking agents that give the stool weight; however, advice must always be given to drink adequate water with these products to avoid obstruction or impaction.

Work by Hardinge and colleagues in 1958, studying crude fibre intake in vegans, omnivores and vegetarians, was confirmed by Burkitt et al. in 1972. It showed that a vegan consumed 23.9 g of fibre a day, a vegetarian 16.3 g and an omnivore 10.7 g. Further studies by Davies and Dickerson (1994) suggested that not only is fibre intake in vegans and vegetarians higher, but also these groups have an improved bowel habit. Although there is an alteration in obtaining energy in vegetarian diets – from carbohydrate because fat is decreased within the diet – those who are vegans need to plan diets carefully so that nutritional status is not compromised.

In balancing good health, dietary fibre should include products that are wholegrain, with five to eleven servings of starchy foods that are wholemeal or wholegrain. NSPs should be from a mixed source such as wholegrain cereals and vegetables with at least five portions of fruit and vegetables per day and two portions of high-fibre cereal per day.

Food labelling for the consumer

For the consumer shopping and organizing meal plans for a family or singleton, understanding what is the 'right' fibre to eat can highlight the practical difficulties of interpreting food labels, although many consumers will be concerned about possible side effects of suddenly increasing fibre intake.

In 1998, the MAFF advised that, for the purpose of food labelling, fibre be defined as NSP in line with COMA's recommendations and that claims relating to fibre should also be based on this definition and on COMA's recommendation of a DRV of 18 g/day. In raising the fibre intake in the diet, there can be potential side effects in the first few months. These can be excessive wind, bloating and abdominal cramps which will gradually lessen, with many patients and consumers finding that constipation is relieved and that it is worth carrying on with the increased fibre intake. In increasing the fibre intake in the diet there are some points that should be followed:

- *The Balance of Good Health* (Health Education Authority, 1996) can provide a plan to follow to develop a well-balanced diet. A start is to move towards consuming more fruit, vegetables, breakfast cereal, potatoes, pasta, rice and bread.
- Consuming more NSPs can be easily organized by eating the correct breakfast cereals which should be wholegrain or bran enriched. Many people do not have breakfast or find that they do not have the time to eat breakfast. Although breakfast is an important meal and more encouragement should be made for people to start the day with a good breakfast, cereal can be eaten at any time of day and often people find that they can eat cereal in the evening before bedtime. Whatever time of day cereal is eaten, it can only help in the uptake of NSPs in the diet. The increase of NSPs in the diet should be done slowly over a period of time to avoid too much gastrointestinal disturbance.
- When fibre in the diet is increased, the fluid intake should increase correspondingly, drinking six to eight cups of water per day along with other fluid that is consumed normally. Most people drink inadequate amounts of water every day and often inadequate amounts of fluid in general, which can lead to headaches and constipation.

High-fibre choices

- Breads: wholegrain breads, muffins, bagels, wheatgerm, oatmeal, wholewheat crackers, wholewheat pasta, brown rice, pita bread, tortillas, pumpernickel, rye bread, rye crispbread.
- Cereals: Weetabix, Branflakes, Shredded Wheat, cooked barley, cooked bulgar, Fruit and Fibre.

- Fruit: blackberries, dried dates, raspberries, apple, apricots, banana, avocado, cranberries, currants, honeydew melon, prunes, orange, pear, citrus fruits, cherries, papaya, pineapple, strawberries, rhubarb, figs, kiwi fruit, kumquats.
- Vegetables: Brussels sprouts, parsnips, peas, corn, broccoli, cabbage, carrots, green beans, onions, potatoes, spinach, squash, asparagus, sweet potatoes, yam, cauliflower, tomato, turnip, radish, aubergine, green pepper, snow peas.
- Dairy: all kinds of milk, cheese, yoghurt, eggs, ice cream.
- Meat: all meat and poultry.
- Fish: all fish.
- Meat substitutes: garbanzo beans, kidney beans, lentils, lima beans, split peas, pinto beans, baked beans, soya beans, smooth peanut butter.
- Nuts and snacks: wholewheat pretzels, almonds, cashews, walnuts, sunflower seeds, cakes and biscuits made with oatmeal.

Although not exhaustive, the above lists give an idea of which foods are high in fibre for consuming in a fibre-enhanced diet and further discussion on foodstuffs and eating after an attack of diverticulitis can be found in Chapter 12.

- Fluid intake: stress and inactivity in modern lives today also play an important part in bowel activity. Much has been said in the media about becoming a nation of couch potatoes and taking very little sustained exercise. This, along with fast food, can lead not only to obesity but also to constipation. Many people who suffer from constipation are advised to eat more fibre and then find that the constipation worsens. For the fibre to work efficiently, the fibre needs to absorb more water and 2 litres of water a day will help to swell the fibre and form softer stools that are easier to pass.

A recent literature review on the evidence of high-fibre diets in diverticular disease was undertaken by Aldoori and Ryan-Harsham (2002) using Medline. The objective was to review dietary factors associated with diverticular disease, particularly looking at the role of dietary fibre. In looking for quality-of-life evidence the author was concentrating on the relationship between dietary factors and other lifestyle factors in diverticular disease. In the literature review using publications from January 1996 to December 2001, 30 references were recorded and many of the articles were either focused on dietary intervention in treating symptomatic cases or case-control studies that had limitations in studying diverticular disease and diet associations. Only one large prospective study, undertaken in the USA in 1998, attempted to assess diet at entry into the study before the diagnosis of diverticular disease. The main message from the review was that a diet high in fibre made up of fruit and vegetables with little fat and red meat decreases the risk of diverticular disease. It appears that the insoluble component of fibre is strongly associated with a lower risk of developing diverticular disease. Caffeine and alcohol do not appear to increase the risk of diverticular disease substantially.

The general conclusion from the literature search confirms much of today's current thinking about diet and diverticular disease – that a food intake that is high in fibre and low in total fat and red meat, a higher fluid intake and more physical activity may help to prevent diverticular disease.

Chapter 12
Alternative Treatments

Complementary therapies or alternative therapies are terms that people use to cover a wide range of non-biomedical interventions to treat sickness and illness. Both patients and healthcare practitioners have preconceived ideas about patterns of illness and how illness should be interpreted and treated. Kleinman (1980) describes the core points that people use to understand and explain their episode of sickness and these core points are known as explanatory models, which help people make decisions in relation to their care and treatment:

- Culturally construct illness as a psychosocial experience
- Establish general criteria to guide the health-seeking process and to evaluate the treatment approach
- Manage particular illness episodes by communication, labelling and explaining
- Engage in healthy activities and therapeutic interventions, medicine, surgery, healing rituals and counselling
- Manage the therapeutic outcome and appropriate treatments for the condition.

The clinical process is one way for the patient to adapt to certain worrying circumstances such as the formation of a stoma, and the cultural construction of an illness can often be a personal and social adaptive response. Illness is the shaping of disease into behaviour and experience that is created by personal, social and cultural reactions to the disease. By asserting the complementary nature of mind and body, healing and curing, Kleinman and his associates reject the crude Cartesianism of the biomedical model of sickness (Young, 1982).

Explanatory models of illness are not new to western biomedicine and practitioners of healing have existed as long as professional functions have been specialized in human society, with medical lore being integral to every existing human culture (Leslie, 1976). Comparisons of the healer or medicine man within a culture have to be understood in a cultural context. Healers have often been called to the role by personal experience; they have acquired arcane knowledge and are deemed to have great powers. Their principal social function is to diagnose and prescribe ritual actions to overcome illness or form a prognosis. As all beliefs are culture bound, little sense can be made of them out of context. They will also change as the society in which they exist changes and newer beliefs displace, merge or coexist with the society's older beliefs. The lay explanatory model is put together in response to a particular episode of illness and is not the same as the individual's general beliefs about illness that his or her society may hold. By contrast, the physician's explanatory model is based on scientific logic and deals with a single cause. Doctor and patient, each using his or her explanatory model, must agree about the interpretation of the model, the individual's subjective view of the illness and the doctor's view of the disease process. Any problems must be resolved by negotiation so that the patient will comply with the prescribed treatment.

Caring and Curing

In most societies when people become ill or suffer discomfort there are often many ways that they may seek help. The more complex a society, the more therapeutic options there are available, most of which need to be paid for. Therefore, western and non-western modern urbanized societies are likely to demonstrate medical pluralism. In the UK there are a wide range of therapeutic options available for the relief of physical discomfort and these fall into three sectors:

- popular sector
- folk sector
- professional sector.

Often these therapeutic options are based on different premises and arise in different cultures, and yet they coexist and may even overlap each other. An example of this coexistence would be acupuncture, which is Chinese in origin and, in China, the use and availability of western medicine. Often it is more the efficacy of the treatment that is important to the patient who is experiencing discomfort rather than the knowledge of the origins of the treatment.

The Popular Sector

This is the area of the layperson who is not a specialist or professional, and it is often in this area that ill-health is first recognized. This sector includes all the therapeutic options available to the public that do not require payment or consultation with medical practitioners or folk healers. This area mainly includes self-medication, and a study by Dunnell and Cartwright in 1972 found that the use of self-prescribed medication was twice as common as the use of prescribed drugs. Self-medication was often used as an alternative to arranging an appointment to see the GP. Laxatives and aspirin are the most common self-prescribed drugs. Often the exchange of medication happens when someone who has been prescribed a drug or is taking a non-prescribed drug for abdominal pain that they found to work for them will offer this to a friend or neighbour who is exhibiting much the same symptoms. Hindmarsh (1981) termed this phenomenon 'over the fence physicians'. The influence of taking or not taking prescribed drugs is part of the popular health culture; it is influenced by lay evaluation of 'does this drug and what it will do make sense?' and this 'reasoning' affects compliance and non-compliance.

One very important area of the popular healthcare sector is the ever-expanding role of self-help groups, which have multiplied many-fold since World War II. In 1982 it was reported that there were about 355 self-help groups in the UK with many thousands of members (Helman, 1990). Most of the categories of self-help groups often overlap and Levy (1982) found that, although many self-help groups were for members who were afflicted and others were for the carers of those afflicted, other self-help groups would be made up of the afflicted and of doctors, nurses and pharmaceutical companies. Self-help groups often start because people feel that existing services in the biomedical area either are not suitable or do not exist, or because like-minded people recognize the value of mutual help. Self-help groups in ostomy care have evolved since the 1930s to help and support the patient with a stoma. Reissman (1965) described the helper therapy principle, implying that it is the helper who may benefit most from the helping role.

In 1963 a pilot scheme was organized at the Royal Marsden Hospital with funding from the King's Fund to establish whether there was a need for some form of group or association for patients who had undergone surgery and had a colostomy. After the initial pilot survey in London, a decision was taken to establish a charity for the purpose of providing guidance and assistance to colostomy patients in the UK, to help with rehabilitation and to enable them to have a better quality of life. The association became a registered charity in 1966 and is now known as the British Colostomy Association. Often those with 'stigmatized' conditions who feel marginalized within their community and society find that 'belonging' to a self-help group or organization helps them to explain and cope with their situation.

The Folk Sector

The folk sector is an ill-defined area with its 'practitioners' aiming at holistic treatment of their patient. Such 'practitioners are faith healers, herbalists, clairvoyants, and the forms of diagnosis and healing are to be found in complementary and alternative medicine, with as many as 13% of the population seeking help from a complementary or alternative therapist every year' (Fulder, 1988). The herbal practitioner believes that disease is an imbalance of the physiological/mental/emotional well-being of the body. The Community Health Foundation considers that the definition of health is not just when there is an absence of pain and discomfort, but that wellness is a relationship between that person and his or her family, friends, environment and working life.

Before the Midwives Act of 1902, when midwifery became registerable, it was considered part of the folk sector along with faith healing and herbalism. The earliest description of the use of herbal remedies can be traced back to AD 1260 (Sharpe, 1979), although it is known that the Egyptians as far back as 1600 BC were using garlic, fennel and thyme. Nicholas Culpeper (1616–1654), an English physician, started to practise astrology and physic in 1640 and in 1649 published an English translation of the *College of Physicians Pharmacopoeia, A Physical Directory*. In 1653 he published *The English Physician Enlarged* also known as the *Herbal*. Both books sold well, with the latter forming the basis of herbalism in the English-speaking world. Although herbs can be used to alleviate various symptoms of illness and help well-being, they can have side effects and interact with other treatments or prescribed or non-prescribed medication.

The folk sector also includes secular and spiritual healers, with spiritual healers describing their practice as laying on of hands, prayer or meditation, whether or not the patient is present. The NHS recognizes that some of their patients may request a spiritual healer and have an agreement in more than 1500 NHS hospitals for the healing member to attend if so requested (Helman, 1990).

Christian Hahnemann (1755–1843) was a German physician and founder of homeopathy; he practised medicine for 10 years. After several years experimenting with bark to understand its curative powers, he came to the conclusion that medicine produces a very similar condition in a healthy person to that which it relieves in the sick. The first homeopathic hospital in the UK was founded in London in 1849. In 1948 the homeopathic hospitals were incorporated into the NHS. Doctors qualified in the allopathic way take postgraduate education in homeopathy and staff the hospitals. Homeopathy in the UK is recognized as a safe alternative therapy as opposed to other forms of alternative medicine and healing. It spans both the folk sector and the professional sector. Other forms of alternative healing have been organized into associations with registers of accredited practitioners such as:

- Osteopathic Medical Association
- Chiropractic Medical Association
- British Acupuncture Association
- Society of Homeopaths
- National Institute of Medical Herbalists
- British Society of Medical and Dental Hypnosis.

Over recent years the interest in alternative and complementary therapies has escalated as people try to find help for illness in other areas, often as a result of their disillusionment with the NHS and long waiting lists. The Institute for Complementary Medicine maintains a register of trained practitioners and organizations affiliated to it. In 1989 the Institute estimated that there were at least 15 000 alternative practitioners in the UK, and these included spiritual healers, osteopaths, acupuncturists, massage practitioners, hypnotherapists, nutritionists, chiropracters, reflexologists and aromatherapists (Helman, 1990). It has been estimated that as many as 75% of abnormal symptoms are treated within the popular and folk sectors of health care (Wadsworth et al., 1971).

Ayurvedic Medicine

Ayurveda is a traditional Hindu system of medicine practised in India and parts of the Far East based on balance in bodily systems and placing emphasis on diet, herbal treatment and yogic breathing. Within the Ayurvedic system, there are complex concepts of the physiology of the body which are believed to help equate health and balance. It is believed that the five elements – ether, wind, water, fire and earth – are the elements that make up life including the three humours and the seven components of the body. Optimal working of the body comes from a balance of the humours and illness from an excess or deficiency of them. Food is used as a means of reducing excess humours and there are 'heat-producing' foods and foods that are 'cooling'. Humoral theory, also known as the hot/cold theory, suggests that health is balanced by the effect of hot and cold on the body. These symbolic powers, not actual temperatures, are believed to be present in food, herbs and medicines, and health returns once the internal temperature balance is re-established.

Although Ayurvedic medicine is more common in the USA than in the UK, it is possible that a herbal prescription could precipitate a flare-up of diverticular disease in a susceptible person using a powerful bowel-cleansing routine. When there is a flare-up of diverticular disease causing abdominal pain and discomfort, Ayurvedic practitioners recommend massaging sesame seed oil into the skin over the stomach and bowel area in the morning and evening.

Acupuncture

Acupuncture is a method of treating various conditions by pricking the skin or tissues with sterile needles. It has been practised in China for more than 4500 years and is increasingly popular in western societies. In 80% of people who have acupuncture there is alleviation from the pain or discomfort. It is thought that acupuncture re-balances the imbalance of the body's condition, with the needles possibly stimulating endorphins, which are naturally occurring pain-killers.

Aromatherapy

Aromatherapy is massage using aromatic plant extracts and essential oils and has become increasingly popular in the western world. As with herbalism, it is believed that plants have healing properties and their scent can affect mood and stress levels. Aromatherapy massage brings together two areas, the scent of the plants being used in massage oil and the touch of the masseuse. Although the true termination of therapeutic touch is in the realm of healing, where the healer holds his or her hands over the afflicted area without actual contact with the body, in aromatherapy it is recognized that touch in massage has a therapeutic value.

Reflexology

Reflexology is a system of massage through reflex points on the feet to relieve tension and help illness. Other areas that can be used are the head and hands, but it is most commonly the feet that are used. Foot massage came from China and originated there over 5000 years ago. Different parts of the body and body organs are aligned to areas on the soles of the feet and treatment is by pressure and massage. Again, it is often the combined pressure and massage associated with therapeutic touch that helps the patient to relax and the gut to cease spasmodic action.

Herbs that may help

Certain herbs as an infusion or in food may help with the symptoms of diverticular disease, especially when there is a flare-up of diverticulitis.

To help the digestion

- Mint, ginger or fennel tea
- Honey
- Comfrey
- Camomile
- Rosemary
- Marshmallow
- Lemon balm
- Peppermint
- Basil
- Aloe vera (not in pregnancy)

Constipation

- Tamarind
- Yellow dock (not in pregnancy)
- Root ginger
- Senna pods

Inflammation

- Parsley
- Aloe vera (not in pregnancy)
- Burdock (not in pregnancy)

Flatulence

- Cinnamon (not in pregnancy)
- Angelica
- Fennel
- Peppermint
- Sage

The types of complementary or alternative therapies that may specifically help in diverticular disease are:

- herbalism
- massage
- acupuncture

- naturopathy
- homoeopathy
- aromatherapy
- reflexology
- yoga
- relaxation therapy
- Ayurveda.

Even though these therapies may offer the patient help or relief from symptoms, they do not replace western orthodox medicine when there are associated complications in diverticular disease, such as haemorrhage, fistula, obstruction and abscess.

Often daily ingestion of 'live bacteria' in the form of *Acidophilus*, *Bifidus* and *Lactobacillus*, in yoghurt, yoghurt drinks (Actimel, etc.) or capsule form, will alleviate the symptoms of flatulence and discomfort after a meal. The action of the live bacteria is to help prevent the unwanted bad bacteria infesting the gut, which can happen if antibiotics have been taken for a flare-up of diverticulitis.

Often constipation aggravates diverticular disease and GPs will prescribe isphagula husk (Fybogel) although it is often not effective and contains additives. A natural way to help the bowel work is to have fruit, particularly papaya, prunes or figs, mixed with cereal or porridge. Herbal tea infusions also help. Pure bran should not be added to food because it is very hard for the gut to break it down (see Chapter 11). If the gut is sensitive during or after an attack of diverticulitis or there is infection or bleeding from the rectum, bland food such as chicken and fish and plain pasta and plenty of water to drink will help until symptoms subside. Red meat, fatty foods and pastries should be avoided. Often the removal of wheat-based products and dairy products from the diet gives some relief and along with caffeine-based drinks and fizzy drinks can bring long-term relief.

In a Danish study (Tonnesen et al., 1999) investigation was made between the association of alcohol and diverticulitis. The study followed a large cohort of men and women discharged from the hospital with the diagnosis of alcoholism between 1977 and 1993. The risk period was defined as from the date of admission to the first hospital diagnosis of diverticulitis, to death or to the end of 1993.

It appears that the risk of diverticulitis was significantly increased in people with alcohol problems, with it being slightly higher in women than in men. Although the aetiology of diverticulitis is unknown, it may be that immunocompromising mechanisms are important. It is known that alcohol can suppress the immune capacity and may be relevant in the risk of diverticulitis in those who abuse alcohol. It is known that ethanol can suppress a variety of T-cell-dependent processes. Other factors often related to alcoholism are malnutrition and smoking. The outcome of the study postulated that the high incidence of diverticulitis may be another complication of alcohol abuse, with increased postoperative morbidity when surgical intervention is needed.

Chapter 13
Current Thinking

As has been seen, diverticular disease is common in the western world and can carry a significant morbidity. Although diverticular disease is common, it is still poorly understood and recent advances in the field continue to focus on the technological side (Cima and Young-Fadok, 2001). Improved computed tomography (CT) allows diagnosis and assessment to be made of severe acute diverticular disease and specialized teams using advanced endoscopic techniques are able to control diverticular bleeding, thereby removing the need for surgical intervention. As yet there are few randomized controlled trials to examine the evidence looking at this approach.

The Scientific Committee of the European Association for Endoscopic Surgery reported on their consensus development conference with the aim of resolving the current controversy over the diagnosis and treatment of diverticular disease (Kohler et al., 1999). A multidisciplinary team of international experts was convened to take part in the consensus exercise. Beforehand the panel was asked to reply to a series of questions on diverticular disease and the consensus statement from these questionnaires was modified at a joint meeting of the panel of experts. These were then presented at the public discussion and again revised by the convened panel of experts.

Using the Delphi method the final consensus was agreed with all the panel members. Asymptomatic diverticulosis, complicated diverticular disease and diverticular disease with actual or recurrent symptoms were all defined in separate categories. As an initial diagnostic tool there was no agreement about whether barium enema or colonoscopy was the better choice as a diagnostic tool in uncomplicated cases. CT is recommended in complicated cases for definitive diagnosis and, after two attacks of diverticular disease, elective surgical intervention should be considered. For those patients with complications, such as bleeding, stenosis and fistula, surgery is also indicated.

The mortality, morbidity and formation of a stoma appear to be dependent on whether the surgery is done by a specialist colorectal surgeon or a general surgeon. In addition the grade of surgeon operating can determine morbidity, mortality and stoma formation (Zorcolo et al., 2003). In the Edinburgh study it was concluded that primary anastomosis for diverticular disease can be performed with low morbidity and mortality in selected patients, thereby reducing the need for a Hartmann's procedure and colostomy, and the subsequent surgery for reversal and closure of the colostomy that can have high complication rates.

Faecal loading and faecal peritonitis do not preclude a primary anastomosis and the main factors contributing to favourable outcomes are the absence of concurrent disease and the patient's general health. Elderly patients who have a high American Society of Anesthesiologists (ASA) score were associated in this study with poorer outcomes.

Does diverticular disease affect the quality of life (QoL) of patients with long-standing symptoms? In a study by Bolster and Papagrigoriadis (2003) their literature search revealed that there were no QoL research studies into diverticular disease and that such studies would be of use in the selection of patients for elective surgical intervention. Structured interviews and questionnaires were given to 100 people, divided into two groups of 50. Group 1 had a diagnosis of diverticular disease with symptoms, and group 2 were well volunteers. The areas of QoL that were looked at were:

- emotional symptoms
- systemic symptoms
- bowel symptoms
- social function.

Scores in group 1 fell significantly behind those in group 2. Particular areas were bowel symptoms and emotional symptoms and all those in group 1 with diverticular disease scored significantly lower on all the QoL areas examined, compared with group 2. The authors believe that diverticular disease does affect a person's QoL and that further research is required so that a tool can be developed that would accurately measure the subjective health status of patients with diverticular disease; this would enable a systematic approach to the delivery of treatment and management of the patient with diverticular disease.

The Evidence

An important aspect in medicine today is the concept of controlled clinical trials and evidence-based medicine. Evidence-based medicine enables the practitioner to assess the scientific validity and practical relevance of articles that are read, and if appropriate, put the results into practice. These are the constituents of the skills needed for evidence-based medicine.

The definition of evidence-based medicine is:

> . . . the conscientious, explicit and judicious use of current best evidence in making decisions about the care of individual patients.
>
> (Sackett et al., 1996)

In deciding the best treatment for diverticular disease information needs to be converted into questions that can be answered:

- Find with maximum efficiency the best evidence, which can be from clinical examination, diagnostics, published literature or other sources.
- The evidence needs to be appraised critically to assess validity and applicability.
- Finally, implementation of the search needs to be used in the clinical practice and the performance evaluated.

The best international source regarding evidence on the effects of common clinical interventions in diverticular disease is available in *Clinical Evidence Concise* (BMA, 2003). This summarizes the current state of knowledge and uncertainties about the prevention and treatment of clinical conditions, based on thorough searches and appraisal of the literature describing the best available evidence from systematic reviews and randomized controlled trials (RCTs).

The most recent evidence for the treatment of uncomplicated diverticular disease from systematic searches in October 2002 is divided into sections.

Likely to be beneficial

- The use of Rifaxamin with glucomannan or glucomannan alone.

One RCT found that oral Rifaxamin with glucomannan versus glucomannan plus a placebo significantly increases the proportion of patients with uncomplicated diverticular disease who are symptom free after 12 months of treatment.

Unknown effectiveness

- Two small RCTs found no consistent effect of bran or isphagula husk versus placebo on symptom relief after 12–16 weeks.
- There are no RCTs of elective or laparoscopic colonic resection.
- One RCT found no significant difference with lactulose versus high-fibre

diet in the number of people who considered themselves to be much improved after 12 weeks.

- One small RCT found no significant difference with methylcellulose versus placebo in mean symptom score after 3 months.

What are the effects of treatments to prevent complications of diverticular disease?

Unknown effectiveness

- Increased fibre intake.

No RCTs were found of advice to consume a high-fibre diet or of dietary fibre supplements.

Trade-off between benefits and harm

One RCT found that mesalazine reduced symptomatic recurrence compared with no treatment in patients previously treated for an episode of acute diverticulitis, but was associated with abdominal pain.

What are the effects of treatments for acute diverticulitis?

Unknown effectiveness

There were no RCTs of medical treatment versus placebo. One RCT comparing intravenous cefoxitin versus intravenous gentamicin plus intravenous clindamycin found no significant difference in rates of clinical cure. Observational studies in patients with acute diverticulitis have found low mortality rates with medical treatment, but that the recurrence rate may be high.

Surgery (for diverticulitis complicated by generalized peritonitis)

There were no RCTs of surgery versus either surgery or medical treatment. One RCT was found that compared the acute resection versus non-acute resection of the sigmoid colon and found no difference in mortality. A second RCT that compared primary versus secondary sigmoid colonic resection found no significant difference in mortality, but did find that primary resection significantly reduced rates of postoperative peritonitis and emergency reoperation.

Conclusion

In current thinking the authors have attempted to give the best evidence that was available at the time of writing. Use of the best clinical evidence, research and systematic searches (*Clinical Evidence Concise*: BMA, 2003) allows the best evidence to be shown for anyone making decisions about patient care. Discussion of current RCTs and information about current effectiveness of various interventions in diverticular disease have been searched for by using explicit methodology to identify gaps in evidence, the effectiveness of various treatments and the benefits versus harm in related treatments. In January 2003, the Association of Coloproctology of Great Britain and Ireland set up an audit into diverticular disease, the National Complications of Diverticular Disease Audit, and has invited all surgeons across the UK to participate as an online database.

Glossary

ACCT air contrast computed tomography.

Aetiology the cause of a condition or disease.

Amino acids form the chief structural components of proteins and are needed in human nutrition.

Anaemia a deficiency in the number of red blood cells in the body, which means that not enough oxygen reaches the tissues and organs.

Barium enema a suspension of barium inserted into the rectum and retained while radiological examination is carried out.

Benign not cancerous.

Biopsy removal of a small piece of tissue from the body for examination under a microscope for diagnosis.

Caecum first part of the large bowel.

Colon part of the large intestine that extends from the caecum to the rectum.

Colonoscopy examination of the colon with an endoscope.

Colorectal to do with the colon or rectum.

Colostomy diversion from the colon on to the abdominal wall to allow the passage of faeces.

Constipation infrequent or difficult evacuation of faeces.

CT computed tomography, the use of X-ray beams to create a three-dimensional image of the body.

Diarrhoea abnormally frequent and liquid faecal discharge.

Diverticulum a protrusion of the inner lining of the intestine through the outer muscular coat to form a small pouch with a narrow neck.

Diverticula more than one diverticulum.

Diverticular pertaining to diverticulum

Diverticulosis the presence of diverticula.

Diverticulitis inflammation of one or more diverticula.

Fistula an abnormal passage between two internal organs.

Hartmann's procedure surgical procedure to divide the colon closing the distal end and bringing the proximal end onto the abdominal wall as a colostomy.

Hot biopsy biopsy forceps attached to an electrocoagulation snare handle.

Laparotomy a surgical incision made through the abdomen.

Laparoscopy examination of the interior of the abdomen using a laparoscope.

Laparoscope a fibreoptic instrument that permits inspection of the peritoneal cavity.

Obstruction a blockage in the bowel.

Perforation a hole made through a body part.

Peristalsis wavelike contractions of the muscle through the bowel.

Proctoscopy inspection of the rectum with a tubular instrument that is illuminated.

Radiologist a doctor who interprets radiographs.

Sigmoid colon the S-shaped part of the colon lying in the pelvis.

Sigmoidoscopy examination of the sigmoid colon with the use of an endoscope.

Stoma artificial opening onto the abdomen to divert faeces or urine.

Stoma nurse a specialist expert nurse who looks after people with stomas.

Stricture a narrowing of a canal or duct.

Villus intestinal villi are the numerous thread-like projections that cover the mucosa of the colon and serve as sites of absorption of fluid and nutrients.

Information and support

British Colostomy Association
BCA Office
13 Station Road
Reading
Berkshire RG1 1LG
Tel: 0118 939 1537
Helpline: 0800 328 4257 – 24 hours
Email: sue@bcass.org.uk
Website: www.bcass.org.uk

British Nutrition Foundation
High Holborn House
52–54 High Holborn
London WC1V 6RQ
Tel: 020 7404 6504
Email: postbox@nutrition.org.uk
Website: www.nutrition.org.uk

Digestive Disorders Foundation
Email: ddf@digestivedisorders.org.uk
Website: www.digestivedisorders.org.uk

Stoma care nurse
Via the switchboard at your local hospital.
Website: www.west-london-scn.co.uk

National Association for Diverticular Disease
7 Cambridge Road
Orrell
Wigan WN5 8PL
Tel: 01942 213572
Email: Ronhop@freenetname.co.uk
Website: www.users.globalnet.co.uk

British Society of Gastroenterology
3 St Andrew's Place
Regents Park
London NW1 4LB
Tel: 020 7486 0341
Email: bsg@mailbox.ulcc.ac.uk
Website: www.bsg.org.uk

USA

American Digestive Health Foundation
7th Floor, 7910 Woodmont Avenue
Bethesda, MD 20814-3015, USA
Tel: + 1 (301) 654 2635
Email: dlee@gastro.org

Canada

Northwestern Society of Intestinal Research
c/o Vancouver Hospital and Health Sciences Centre
855 W. 12th Avenue
Vancouver
BC V5Z 1M9, Canada
Tel: + 1 (604) 875 4875
Email: nsir@interchange.ubc.ca

Australia

Gastroenterology Society of Australia
145 Macquarie St
Sydney
NSW 2000, Australia
Tel: +61 2 9256 5454
Website: www.gesa.org.au

References

Abrams JS (1984) Abdominal Stomas. Boston: John Wright.

Aldoori W, Ryan-Harsham M (2002) Preventing diverticular disease. Review of recent evidence on high fibre diets. Canadian Family Physician 48: 1632-7.

Aldoori WH, Giovanucci EL, Rimm ER et al. (1995) Prospective study of physical activity and the risk of symptomatic diverticular disease in men. Gut 36: 276-82.

Aldoori WH, Giovaucci EL, Rockett HR, Sampson L, Rimm EB, Willett WC (1998) A prospective study of dietary fibre types and symptomatic diverticular disease in men. Journal of Nutrition 128: 714-19.

Almy TP, Howell DA (1980) Diverticular disease of the colon. New England Journal of Medicine 302: 324-31.

Ambrosetti P, Robert JH, Witzig JA, Mirescu D, Mathey P, Borst F (1994) Acute left colonic diverticulitis in young patients. Journal of the American College of Surgeons 179: 156-60.

Anderson DN, Driver CP, Davidson AI, Keenan RA (1997) Diverticular disease in patients under the age of fifty. Journal Royal College Surgeons, Edinburgh 42: 102-4.

Arfwidsson S (1964) Pathogenesis of multiple diverticula of the sigmoid colon in diverticular disease. Acta Chirurgica Scandinavica Supplement 342.

Bär A (1993) Definition of Dietary Fibre for Nutritional Labelling Purposes. Binningen, Switzerland: Bioresco AG.

Basse L, Hjort Jakobsen D, Billesbolle P, Werner M, Kehlet H (2000) A clinical pathway to accelerate recovery after colonic resection. Annals of Surgery 232: 51-7.

Bassotti G, Chistolini F, Morelli A (2003) Pathophysiological aspects of diverticular disease of the colon and the role of large bowel motility. World Journal of Gastroenterology 10: 2140-2.

Beer E (1904) Some pathological and clinical aspects of acquired (false) diverticula of the intestine. American Journal of Medical Science 128: 135.

Bell FG (1929) Diverticulitis. Journal College Surgeons, Australia ii: 226-32.

Belmonte C, Klas JV, Perez JJ, Wong WD, Rothenberger DA, Goldberg SM (1996) The Hartmann Procedure. First choice or last resort in diverticular disease. Archives of Surgery 131: 612-15.

Berry CS, Fearn T, Fisher N, Gregory JA, Hardy J (1984) Dietary fibre and prevention of diverticular disease of the colon: evidence from rats. Lancet ii: 294.

Bingham SA, Pett S, Day KC (1990) Non starch polysaccharide intake of a representative sample of British adults. Journal of Human Nutrition and Dietetics 3: 333-7.

Biondo S, Perea MT, Rague JM, Pares D, Jaurrieta E (2001) One stage procedure in non elective surgery for diverticular disease complications. Colorectal Disease 3: 42–5.

Biondo S, Pares D, Rague J, Kreisler E, Fraccalvieri D, Jaurriete E (2002) Acute colonic diverticulitis in patients under 50 years of age. British Journal Surgery 89: 1137–41.

Black P (1987) The appliance of science. Community Outlook May.

Black P (1990) Stoma care in the community. Nursing Standard 4(43): 54–5.

Black P (1992) Body image after enterostomal therapy. Unpublished MSc thesis, Steinberg Collection. London: Royal College of Nursing.

Black P (1994) Management of patients undergoing stoma surgery. British Journal of Nursing 3: 211–16.

Black P (1995) Stoma care: finding the appropriate appliance. British Journal of Nursing 4: 188–92.

Black P (1996) Stoma appliances: what's new? Nurse Prescriber/Community Nurse, April.

Black P (1997) Practical stoma care. A community approach. British Journal of Community Health Nursing 2: 249–53.

Black P (2000) Holistic Stoma Care. London: Ballière Tindall.

BMA (2003) Clinical Evidence Concise 10. London: BMJ Publishing Group.

Bolster LT, Papagrigoriadis S (2003) Diverticular disease has an impact on the quality of life – results of a preliminary study. Colorectal Disease 5: 320–3.

Breckman B (1981) Stoma Care. Beaconsfield: Beaconsfield Publishers.

Brodribb AJM, Humphreys DM (1976) Diverticular disease: three studies. Part 2, Treatment with bran. British Medical Journal i: 425–8.

Bruce CJ, Coller JA, Murray JJ, Schoetz DJ, Roberts PL, Rusin LC (1996) Laparoscopic resection for diverticular disease. Diseases of the Colon and Rectum 39(10): 51–6.

Burkitt DP, Trowell HC (eds) (1975) Refined Carbohydrate Foods and Disease. Some implications of dietary fibre. London: Academic Press.

Burkitt DP, Clements JL, Eaton SB (1985) Prevalence of diverticular disease, hiatus hernia and pelvic phleboliths in black and white Americans. Lancet ii: 880–1.

Burkitt DP, Walker ARP, Painter NS (1972) Effect of dietary fibre on stools and transit times, and its role in the causation of disease. Lancet ii: 1408–12.

Chang WYM (1965) Diverticulitis in Hawaii. Hawaii Medical Journal 24: 442–5.

Chia JG, Chintana C, Wilde MD et al. (1991) Trends of diverticular disease of the large bowel in a newly developed country. Disease of Colon and Rectum 34: 498–501.

Cima RR, Young-Fadok TM (2001) New developments in diverticula disease. Current Gastroenterology Reports 3: 420–4.

Cohen F (1975) Psychological preparation, coping and recovery from surgery. In: Stone GC, Cohen F, Adler NE (eds), Health Psychology. London: Jossey-Bass.

Cohen F, Lazarus RS (1973) Active coping processes, coping dispositions and recovery from surgery. Psychosomatic Medicine 35: 375–89.

Cohen F, Lazarus R (1982) Coping with the stress of illness. In: Stone GC (ed.), Health Psychology. London: Jossey-Bass.

Coode PE, Chan KW, Chai YT (1985) Polyps and diverticula of the large intestine: a necropsy survey in Hong Kong. Gut 26: 1045–8.

CORCE (1997) Stoma Siting. Maidenhead, Berkshire: Medical Projects International.

Cummings JH, Stephen AM (1980) Mechanism of action of dietary fibre in the human colon. Nature 284: 283–4.

Davidson SS, Passmore R (1979) Human Nutrition and Dietetics. Edinburgh: Churchill Livingstone.

Davies J (1999) The right fibre for the right disease. In: Hill M (ed.), International Congress and Symposium Series 236. London: Royal Society of Medicine Press Ltd.

Davies GJ, Dickerson JWT (1994) Bowel function and bowel disease and vegetarianism. South African Medical Journal 84(7): 42–3.

Debray C, Hardouin J, Besancon F, Raimbault J (1961) Frequence de la diverticulose colique selon l'age. Semaine des Hospitaux de Paris 37: 1743. Cited by Painter NS, Burkitt DP (1975) Diverticular disease. Clinical Gastroenterology 4: 3–21.

Department of Health (1991) Dietary Reference Values for Food, Energy and Nutrients for the United Kingdom. Report of the Panel on Dietary Reference Values of the Committee on Medical Aspects of Food Policy. London: HMSO.

Devlin HB (1984) Stomas and stoma care. In: Bouchier IAD, Allan RN, Hodgson HJF, Keighley MRB (eds), Textbook of Gastroenterology. London: Ballière Tindall.

Devlin HB, Plant J, Griffin M (1971) Aftermath of surgery for anorectal cancer. British Medical Journal iii: 413–18.

Dinnick T (1934) The origins and evolution of colostomy. British Journal of Surgery 22: 142–54.

Douglas M (1966) Purity and Danger: An analysis of the concepts of pollution and taboo. Harmondsworth: Penguin.

Dunnell K, Cartwright A (1972) Medicine Takers, Prescribers and Hoarders. A study of self medication in the UK. London: Routledge & Kegan Paul.

Dwivedi A, Chahin F, Agrawal S et al. (2002) Laparoscopic colectomy versus open colectomy for sigmoid diverticular disease. Diseases of the Colon and Rectum 45: 1309–14.

Dyk RB, Sutherland AM (1956) Adaptation of the spouse and other family members to the colostomy patient. Cancer 9: 123–38.

Eastwood MA, Mitchell WD (1976) Mechanism of action of dietary fibre in the human colon. In: Spiller GA, Amen RJ (eds), Fibre in Human Nutrition. New York: Plenum, pp. 109–30.

Ebersole P, Hess P (1998) Towards Healthy Aging. St Louis: Mosby.

Edel M (1894) Ober Erworbene Darmdivertikel. Virchows Archiv für Pathologische Anatomie 138: 347.

Ellis H (1970) Colonic diverticula: pathology and natural history. British Medical Journal iii: 565–7.

Emmett PM, Symes CL, Heaton KW (1993) Dietary intake and sources of non-starch polysaccharide in English men and women. European Journal of Clinical Nutrition 47: 20–30.

Englyst HN, Quigley ME, Hudson GJ (1994) Determination of dietary fibre as non starch polysaccharide with gas liquid chromatographic, high performance liquid chromatographic or spectrophotometric measurement of constituent sugars. Analyst 119: 1497–509.

Englyst HN, Trowell H, Southgate D, Cummings JH (1987) Dietary fibre and resistant starch. American Journal of Clinical Nutrition 46: 873–4.

Erdmann JF (1932) Diverticulitis and diverticulosis. Journal of the American Medical Association xcix: 1125–8.

Findlay JM, Smith AN, Mitchell WD, Anderson AJB, Eastwood MA (1974) Effects of unprocessed bran on colon function in normal subjects and in diverticular disease. Lancet i: 146–9.

Fulder S (1988) Handbook of Complementary Medicine. London: Oxford University Press.

Garry RC (1971) Diet and diverticulosis. British Medical Journal ii: 773.

Gear JSS, Ware A, Fursdon P (1979) Symptomless diverticular disease and intake of dietary fibre. Lancet i: 511–14.

Gill T, Feinstein A (1994) A critical appraisal of the quality of life measurements. Journal of the American Medical Association 272: 619–26.

Goffman E (1963) Stigma. London: Pelican.

Gonzalez R, Smith CD, Mattar SG et al. (2003) Laparoscopic vs open resection for the treatment of diverticular disease. Surgical Endoscopy in press.

Good B (1977) The heart of what's the matter: the semantics of illness in Iran. Culture, Medicine and Psychiatry 1: 25–58.

Green JH (1978) Basic Clinical Physiology. London: Oxford University Press.

Guyatt C, Cook D (1994) Health status, quality of life, and the individual patient. Journal of the American Medical Association 272: 630–1.

Halligan S, Saunders B (2002) Imaging diverticular disease. Clinical Gastroenterology 16: 595–610.

Hardinge MG, Chambers AC, Crooks H et al. (1958) Nutritional studies of vegetarians III. Dietary levels of fibre. American Journal of Clinical Nutrition 6: 523–5.

Hartmann H (1923) Congres Français de Chirurgie 30: 411.

Hartwell JA, Cecil RL (1910) Intestinal diverticula: A pathological and clinical study. American Journal of the Medical Sciences 140: 174–203.

Health Education Authority (1996) The Balance of Good Health. London: HEA.

Heaton K (1985) Diet and diverticulitis – new leads. Gut 22: 541–543.

Helman C (1990) Culture, Health and Illness. London: Wright.

Henderson HP (1994) Diverticulosis and diverticulitis. British Journal of Radiology 17: 197.

Hilden K (1933) Maapallon esihistorialliset ja nykyiset ihmisrodut. Werner Soderstrom: Porvoo.

Hill M (1999) The right fibre for the right disease. International Congress and Symposium series 236. London: Royal Society of Medicine Press.

Hinchey EJ, Schaal PG, Richards GK (1978) Treatment of perforated diverticular disease of the colon. Advances in Surgery 12: 85–109.

Hindmarsh I (1981) Too many pills in the cupboard. New Society 55: 142–3.

Hipsley EH (1953) 'Dietary fibre' and pregnancy toxaemia. British Medical Journal ii: 420–2.

Holland JC, Winter DC, Richardson D (2002) Laparoscopically assisted reversal of Hartmann's procedure revisited. Surgical Laparoscopy Endoscopy and Percutaneous Techniques 12: 291–4.

Horgan AF, McConnell E, Wolff BG, The S, Paterson C (2001) Atypical diverticular disease: surgical results. Diseases of the Colon and Rectum 44: 1315–18.

Horner JL (1958) Natural history of diverticulosis of the colon. American Journal of Digestive Diseases 3: 343–50.

Hughes LE (1969) Post mortem studies of the colon with special reference to diverticular disease. Gut 10: 336–51.

Hyde C (2003) Diverticular disease. Gastrointestinal Nursing 1(5): 34–9.

IMS Hospital Group Ltd (2003) New Stoma Patient Feedback. Kent: Sittingbourne Research Centre.

Jackson S (1979) Anatomy and Physiology for Nurses, 9th edn. London: Ballière Tindall.

Jones S (1859) Transactions of the Pathological Society 10: 131.

Keeley KJ (1958) Alimentary disease in the Bantu – a review. Medical Proceedings, Johannesburg, SA 4: 281–6.

Keighley MR, Williams N (1997) Surgery of the Anus, Rectum and Colon, part 2. London: WB Saunders, pp. 1128–11, 1956–62.

Kelly M (1985) Loss and grief reactions as responses to surgery. Journal of Advanced Nursing 10: 517–25.

Kim EH (1964) Hiatus hernia and diverticulum of the colon: low incidence in Korea. New England Journal of Medicine 271: 764–8.

Klebs E (1869) Handbuch der Pathologischen Anatomie. Berlin: Hirschwald, p. 271.

Kleinman A (1980) Patients and Healers in the Context of Culture. Berkley, CA: University of California Press.

Klopp A (1990) Body image and self concept among individuals with stomas. Journal of Enterostomal Therapy 17: 98-105.

Kohler L, Sauerland S, Neugebauer E (1999) Diagnosis and treatment of diverticular disease: results of a consensus development conference. Surgical Endoscopy 13: 430-60.

Kohler R (1963) The incidence of colonic diverticula in Finland and Sweden. Acta Chirurgica Scandinavica 126: 148-55.

Konvolinka CW (1994) Acute diverticulitis under the age of 40. American Journal of Surgery 167: 562-5.

Krukowski ZH (1998) In: Phillips RKS (ed.), Colorectal Surgery. London: WB Saunders, pp. 123-40.

Kyle J, Adesola AO, Tinckler LF et al. (1967) Incidence of diverticulitis. Scandinavian Journal of Gastroenterology 2: 77-80.

Lambert JP, Dickerson JWT (1989) A survey of high fibre diet sheets used in the treatment of irritable bowel syndrome in Great Britain. Journal of Human Nutrition and Dietetics 2: 429-35.

Larimore JW (1925) Diverticulitis of the large intestine. Journal of the Missouri Medical Association 22: 129.

Leakey AL, Ellis RM, Quill DS, Peel ALG (1985) High fibre diet in symptomatic diverticular disease of the colon. Annals of the Royal College of Surgeons of England 67: 173-4.

Lee YS (1986) Diverticular disease of the large bowel in Singapore: an autopsy survey. Diseases of the Colon and Rectum 29: 330-5.

Leslie C (1976) Asian Medical Systems: A comparative study. Berkley, CA: University of California Press.

Levy L (1982) Mutual support groups in Great Britain. Social Science and Medicine 16: 1265-75.

Lewis SJ, Heaton KW (1997) Stool form scale as a useful guide to intestinal transit time. Scandinavian Journal Gastroenterology 32: 920-4.

Littlewood J (1985) No flag day for incontinence. Self Health September: 32-4.

Littlewood J, Holden P (eds) (1991) Anthropology and Nursing. London: Routledge.

Littre M (1732) Histoire de l'Academie Royale des Sciences. Paris, France, pp. 36-7.

Lockhart-Mummery JP, Hodgson HG (1931) Observations on diverticula of the colon and their sequelae. British Medical Journal i: 525-7.

McConnell AA, Eastwood MA, Mitchell WD (1974) Physical charateristics of vegetable food stuffs that could influence bowel functions. Journal of Science, Food and Agriculture 25: 1457-64.

McConnell EJ, Tessier DJ, Wolff BG (2003) Population based incidence of complicated diverticular disease of the sigmoid colon based on gender and age. Diseases of the Colon and Rectum 46: 1110-14.

Majeed A (1998) Using PACT to audit prescribing of stoma care products. Clinical Care, General Medicine. National Association of Fundholding Practices Yearbook.

Manousos ON, Truelove SC, Lumsden K (1967) Transit time of food in patients with diverticulosis or irritable colon syndrome and normal subjects. British Medical Journal 3(568): 760-2.

Manousos O, Day NE, Tzonoua A et al. (1985) Diet and other factors in the aetiology of diverticulosis: an epidemiological study in Greece. Gut 26: 544-9.

Mayo WJ (1930) Diverticula of the sigmoid. American Surgery 92: 739.

Mimura T, Emanuel A, Kamm MA (2002) Pathophysiology of diverticular disease. Best Practice in Research in Clinical Gastroenterology 16: 563–76.

Ministry of Agriculture, Fisheries and Food (MAFF) (1997) National Food Survey 1996. London: The Stationery Office.

MAFF (1998) Food safety information bulletin. COMA News. Bulletin No. 97, June.

Morrison J (1978) Rehabilitation of the ostomate. Australian Nurses Journal 8: 46–8.

Munakata A, Nakagi S, Toshida Y et al. (1982) Study on the diverticula disease of the colon in Korea. Japanese Society of Coloproctology 35: 224–31.

Ornstein MH, Littlewood ER, Baird IM et al. (1981) Are fibre supplements really necessary in diverticula disease of the colon? A controlled trial. British Medical Journal 282: 1353–6.

Oschner HC, Bargen MD (1935) Diverticulosis of the large intestine: An evaluation of historical and personal observations. Annals of Internal Medicine 9: 282–96.

O'Shea H (2001) Teaching the adult ostomy patient. Journal of Wound Ostomy Continence Nursing 28: 47–54.

Padilla C, Grant M (1985) Quality of Life as a cancer nursing outcome variable. Advances in Nursing Science 8: 45–60.

Painter NS (1964) The aetiology of diverticulosis of the colon with special reference to the action of certain drugs on the behaviour of the colon. Annals of the Royal College of Surgeons of England 34: 98–119.

Painter NS, Burkitt DP (1969) Diverticular disease of the colon: a disease of this century. Lancet ii: 586–8.

Painter NS, Burkitt DP (1971) Diverticular disease of the colon: a deficiency disease of Western civilisation. British Medical Journal ii: 450–4.

Painter NS, Burkitt DP (1975) Diverticular disease of the colon, a 20th century problem. Clinical Gastroenterology 4: 3–21.

Painter NS, Almeida AZ, Colebourne KW (1972) Unprocessed bran in the treatment of diverticular disease of the colon. British Medical Journal ii: 137–40.

Parkes C (1972) Bereavement: Studies of grief in adult life. Harmondsworth: Pelican.

Parks TG (1968) Post mortem studies of the colon with special reference to diverticular disease. Proceedings of Royal Society of Medicine 61: 30.

Plumley PF, Francis B (1973) Dietary management of diverticular disease. Journal of the American Dietetic Association 63: 527–30.

Pringle W, Swan E, Wade B (1997) Continuing care for stoma patients. Paper given to the RCN Stoma Care Forum.

Rankin FW, Brown PW (1930) Diverticulitis of the colon. Surgery, Gynaecology and Obstetrics 50: 836.

Readding L (2003) Stoma siting: what the community nurse needs to know. British Journal of Community Nursing 8: 502–11.

Redman BK (1988) The Process of Patient Education, 6th edn. St Louis: Mosby, pp. 65–80.

Regenet N, Pessaux P, Hennekinne S et al. (2003) Primary anastomosis after intraoperative colonic lavage versus Hartmann procedure in generalised peritonitis complicating diverticular disease of the colon. International Journal of Colorectal Disease 18: 503–7.

Reisman Y, Ziu Y, Kravrovitc D, Negri M, Wolloch Y, Halevy A (1999) Diverticulitis: the effect of age and location on the course of the disease. International Journal Colorectal Disease 14: 250–4.

Reissman F (1965) The 'Leper' therapy principle. Social Work 10: 27–32.

Ripolles T, Agramunt M, Martinez MJ, Costa S, Gomez-Abril SA, Richart J (2003) The role of ultrasound in the diagnosis, management and evolutive prognosis of acute left sided colonic diverticulitis: a review of 208 patients. European Radiology 13: 2587-95.

Rotert H, Noldge G, Encke J, Richter GM, Dux M (2003) The value of CT for the diagnosis of acute diverticulitis. Radiologe 43(1): 51-8.

Rubin P, Devlin B (1987) The quality of life with a stoma. British Journal of Hospital Medicine 38: 3006.

Sackett DL, Rosenberg WMC, Gray JAM (1996) Evidence based medicine: what it is and what it isn't. British Medical Journal 312: 71-2.

Schwesinger WH, Page CP, Gaskill HV (2000) Operative management of diverticular emergencies: strategies and outcomes. Archives of Surgery 135: 558-62.

Segal I, Solomon A, Hunt JA (1977) Emergence of diverticular disease in the Urban South African black. Gastroenterology 72: 215-19.

Sharpe D (1979) The pattern of over the counter 'prescribing'. MIMS Magazine 15 September: 39-45.

Sher ME, Cheney L, Ricciardi J (1999) Diverticular disease. In: Porrett T, Daniel N (eds), Essential Coloproctology. London: Whurr.

Sim GPG, Scobie BA (1982) Large bowel diseases in New Zealand based on 1118 air contrast enemas. New Zealand Medical Journal 95: 611-13.

Smaje C (1995) Health, Race and Ethnicity: Making sense of the evidence. London: King's Fund Institute.

Smith CC, Christensen WR (1959) The incidence of colonic diverticulitis. Journal of Roentgenology 82: 996.

Smithwick RM (1942) Experiences in the surgical management of diverticulitis of the sigmoid. Annals of Surgery 115: 969.

Society of Gastroenterology Nurses and Associates (1998) Gastroenterology Nursing. A core curriculum. St Louis, MI: Mosby Inc.

Sosa JL, Sleeman D, Puente I, McKenney MG, Hartmann R (1994) Laparoscopic assisted colostomy closure after Hartmann's procedure. Disease of the Colon and Rectum 37: 149-52.

Southgate DA, Durnin JV (1970) Calorie conversion factors. An experimental reassessment of the factors used in the calculation of the energy value of human diets. British Journal Nutrition 24: 517-35.

Spivak H, Weinrauch S, Harvey JC, Surick B, Ferstenberg H, Friedman I (1997) Acute colonic diverticulitis in the young. Diseases of Colon and Rectum 40: 570-4.

Spriggs EI, Marxer OA (1925) Intestinal diverticula. Quarterly Journal of Medicine 19: 1.

Spriggs EI, Marxer OA (1927) Multiple diverticular of the colon. Lancet i: 1067-74.

Stemmermann GN (1970) Patterns of disease among Japanese living in Hawaii. Archives of Environmental Health 20: 266-73.

Stephen AM, Cummings JH (1980) Mechanism of action of dietary fibre in the human colon. Nature 284: 283-4.

Stollman NH, Rashkin JB (1999) Diverticular disease of the colon. Journal of Gastroenterology 29: 241-52.

Sugihara K, Muto T, Morioka Y et al. (1984) Diverticular disease of the colon in Japan: a review of 615 cases. Diseases of Colon and Rectum 27: 531-7.

Sullivan A (2000) Healthy eating: something to chew over? Nursing Standard 14(22): 43-6.

Sutherland A, Orbach C, Dyk R et al. (1952) The psychological impact of cancer and cancer surgery. Cancer 5: 857-72.

Taylor I, Duthie HL (1976) Bran tablets and diverticular disease. British Medical Journal i: 425-8.

Telling WHM, Grunner OC (1917) Acquired diverticula, diverticulitis, and peridiverticulitis of the large intestine. British Journal of Surgery 4: 468-530.

Thompson WG, Patel DG (1986) Clinical picture of diverticular disease of the colon. Clinics in Gastroenterology 15: 903-16.

Thompson WG, Patel DG, Tao N, Nair RC (1982) Does uncomplicated diverticular disease produce symptoms? Digestive Disease and Sciences 27: 605-8.

Tonnesen H, Engholm G, Moller H (1999) Association between alcoholism and diverticulitis. British Journal of Surgery 8: 1067-8.

Tortora G, Anagnostakos N (1981) Principles of Anatomy and Physiology, 3rd edn. New York: Harper & Row.

Travis SPL, Taylor RH, Misiewicz JJ (1993) Colonic diverticular disease. In: Gastroenterology. Oxford: Blackwell Scientific Publications.

Trowell HC (1960) Non-infective Diseases in Africa. London: Arnold.

Trowell HC, Southgate DA, Wolever TM et al. (1976) Dietary fibre redefined. Lancet i: 967.

Tudor RG, Farmarkis N, Keighley MR (1994) National audit of complicated diverticular disease: analysis of index cases. British Journal of Surgery 81: 730-2.

Turner V (1967) The Forest of Symbols. Ithaca: Cornell University Press.

US Department of Health, Education and Welfare (1979) Report to the Congress of the United States of the National Commission on Digestive Diseases. Bethesda: DHEW Publication.

Vajrabukka T, Saksornchai K, Jimakorn P (1980) Diverticular disease of the colon in a Far Eastern Community. Diseases of the Colon and Rectum 23: 151-4.

Wade B (1989) A Stoma is for Life. Harrow, Middx: Scutari Press.

Wadsworth MEJ, Butterfield WJH, Blaney R (1971) Health and Sickness: The choice of treatment. London: Tavistock.

West SD, Robinson EK, Delu AN, Ligon RE, Kao LS, Mercer DW (2003) Diverticulitis in the younger patient. American Journal of Surgery 186: 743-6.

White C (1997) Living with a Stoma. London: Sheldon Press.

Wong D, Wexner S (2000) Practice parameters for the treatment of sigmoid diverticulitis: supporting documentation. The Standards Task Force. The American Society of Colon and Rectal Surgeons, pp. 1-15.

Woods RJ, Lavery IC, Fazio VW, Jagleman DG, Weakley FL (1988) Internal fistulas in diverticular disease. Diseases of the Colon and Rectum 31: 591-6.

Young A (1982) The anthropologics of illness and sickness. Annual Review of Anthropology 11: 257-85.

Zorcolo I, Covotts L, Carlomango N, Bartolo DC (2003) Safety of primary anastomosis in emergency colorectal surgery. Colorectal Disease 5: 262-9.

Index

Page numbers in bold type refer to figures. An asterisk (*) before a page number denotes an entry in the glossary